THE
HEART and LUNG
in
OBESITY

Edited by

Martin A. Alpert, MD

Professor of Medicine
Director, Division of Cardiology
University of South Alabama
College of Medicine
Mobile, Alabama

and

James K. Alexander, MD

Professor of Medicine
Baylor College of Medicine
Houston, Texas

Futura Publishing Company
Armonk, New York

Library of Congress Cataloging-in-Publication Data

The heart and lung in obesity / edited by Martin A. Alpert, James K.
Alexander.
    p.   cm.
    Includes bibliographical references and index.
    ISBN 0-87993-685-1
    1. Heart—Diseases. 2. Cardiopulmonary system—Diseases.
3. Obesity—Complications. I. Alpert, Martin A. II. Alexander,
James K., 1920– .
    [DNLM: 1. Obesity—physiopathology. 2. Obesity—complica-
tions. 3. Heart Diseases—complications. 4. Respiratory Tract
Diseases—complications. WD 210 H436 1997]
    RC682.H365   1997
    616.3'9807—dc21
    DNLM/DLC
    for Library of Congress   97-30470
                                                   CIP

Copyright © 1998
Futura Publishing Company, Inc.

Published by
Futura Publishing Company, Inc.
135 Bedford Road
Armonk, New York 10504

LC #: 97-30470
ISBN #: 0-87993-685-1

To my wife Becky, my children Justin and Jason,
and to Leonard Sternberg.

Martin A. Alpert

To my wife Carolyn and my children James Jr., Susan, and Joan.

James K. Alexander

Preface

Obesity is a chronic and costly health problem that has reached epidemic proportions. Based on the Third National Health and Nutrition Examination Survey reported in 1991, obesity is present in at least 35% of American women and 31% of American men, and is thought to be at least as prevalent in most other industrialized nations. Indeed, obesity is now more common than cigarette smoking.

Heightened awareness of the prevalence of obesity has translated into investigative interest in its genetic and pathophysiological mechanisms and has led to an enormous proliferation of publications in obesity-related areas in recent years. With this has come a greater appreciation of the multifaceted biological implications of obesity, especially in relation to endocrine, metabolic, pulmonary, and cardiovascular function. This book is a critical and comprehensive review of the effects of obesity on heart and lung.

To a considerable extent, but by no means exclusively, this book is concerned with the cardiovascular and pulmonary effects of severe or morbid obesity. Although a spectrum of effects maybe defined with varying degrees of obesity on cardiac morphology and function, hypertension, and coronary artery disease, it is with severe or morbid obesity that cardiorespiratory failure may ultimately develop. Thus, the cardiomyopathy of obesity and related pulmonary complications as found in morbid obesity receive special attention.

After a brief chronological review of investigations leading to our current understanding of the cardiopulmonary effects of obesity by Dr. Alexander, an exposition of the effects of obesity on cardiac structure and function and pulmonary function follows. Dr. Schaffer discusses the effects of obesity on myocardial metabolism, morphology and function in the (fa/fa) Zucker rat, an animal model commonly used in the study of obesity. This chapter sets the stage for the next four, which deal with the effects of obesity on cardiac morphology and function in man. Drs. Alpert and Alexander describe the effects of obesity and weight loss on cardiac morphology based on postmortem, myocardial biopsy, and echocardiographic studies. Thereafter, Drs. Alexander and Alpert discuss the central and peripheral hemodynamic alterations associated with obesity at rest, during exercise and after weight loss. Following this, Drs. Chakko, Alpert, and Alexander provide chapters that review the effects of obesity on diastolic and systolic ventricular function at rest, during exercise and after weight loss. In their chapter on obesity, hypertension, and the heart, Drs. Reisen and Cook summarize epidemiological studies relating to incidence and severity and then discuss current concepts regarding obesity hypertension before and after weight reduction. Dr. Rochester follows with a critical and comprehensive discussion of the effects of obesity on pulmonary function with special attention to the obesity hypoventilation syndrome.

The focus of the book then turns to clinical manifestations and treatment. Drs. Alexander and Alpert describe the pathophysiology and clinical manifestations of obesity cardiomyopathy and discuss the value and limitations of noninvasive cardiac tests in the evaluation of obese patients. Drs. Koenig and Suratt provide a comprehensive discussion of obesity and sleep disordered breathing including sections on pathophysiology, clinical manifestations and management. Drs. Alpert and Alexander follow with a chapter on treatment of obesity cardiomyopathy including discussions of the cardiac effects of starvation and very low calorie diets and of appetite suppressant drugs.

Dr. Alexander concludes by devoting considerable attention to the issue of coronary heart disease and obesity in view of the controversies in interpretation of epidemiologic data, the potential interplay of diabetes mellitus and insulin resistance with coronary artery disease in obese subjects, and more recent studies implicating fat tissue distribution and its metabolic consequences in the pathogenesis of coronary artery disease. Correlation of coronary artery pathologic and angiographic studies with obesity is also addressed. This is an area that has previously received little attention in literature.

A brief appendix is included to aid in clarifying terminology of indices used to describe and quantify obesity.

The contents of this book will be of interest to biochemists, physiologists, primary care physicians, cardiologists, pulmonologists, bariatric surgeons, and nutritionists working in the field of obesity or providing medical care to obese patients. This book is designed to be a comprehensive review of the cardiopulmonary effects of obesity, a reference wherein information from disparate sources is brought together under a single cover.

The editors are indebted to Drs. Chakko, Cook, Koening, Reisin, Rochester, and Suratt for their comprehensive and discerning chapters in this book. Their contributions significantly augment coverage of the proposed subject and help to define it.

The editors acknowledge and appreciate the assistance of Myra Evans and Jana Grana in coordinating the efforts of the contributing authors and in preparing the manuscript. We also thank Mr. Stephen Korn, our publisher, for his continued enthusiasm and advice.

Martin A. Alpert, MD
James K. Alexander, MD

Contributors

James K. Alexander, MD
Professor of Medicine, Baylor College of Medicine, Houston, TX

Martin A. Alpert, MD
Professor of Medicine, Director, Division of Cardiology, University of South Alabama College of Medicine, Mobile, AL

Simon M. Chakko, MD
Chief, Non-invasive Cardiology, Miami VAMC, Associate Professor of Medicine, University of Miami, Miami, FL

M. Eileen Cook, MD
Associate Professor of Medicine, Director, Clinical Nephrology, Louisiana State University School of Medicine, New Orleans, LA

Steven M. Koenig, MD
Assistant Professor of Internal Medicine, Sleep Disorders Center, Division of Pulmonary and Critical Care Medicine, University of Virginia School of Medicine, Charlottesville VA

Efrain Reisen, MD
Professor of Medicine, Director, Section of Nephrology, Louisiana State University School of Medicine, New Orleans, LA

Dudley F. Rochester, MD
Professor Emeritus, Department of Medicine, Division of Pulmonary and Critical Care Medicine, University of Virginia, Charlottesville, VA

Stephen W. Schaffer, PhD
Professor of Pharmacology, University of South Alabama, College of Medicine, Mobile, AL

Paul M. Suratt, MD
John L. Guerrant Professor of Internal Medicine, Director Sleep Disorders Center, Division of Pulmonary and Critical Care Medicine, University of Virginia School of Medicine, Charlottesville VA

Contents

Chapter 1

Historical Notes

James K. Alexander, M.D.

In his treatise, *The Story of Fatty Heart. A Disease of Victorian Times,*[1] Bedford reviews pathological studies from as early as 1783 by Senac,[2] which records excess fat deposition in relation to the heart. According to Bedford, Laennec[3] was the first to establish fatty heart as an entity, and to distinguish between surcharge of fat on the surface of the heart and fatty degeneration in which the muscular substance was transformed into fat exhibiting a yellowish pallor like dead leaves. Quain[4] and his contemporaries followed Laennec in distinguishing between fatty surcharge over the heart surface, especially the right ventricle (RV), and fatty degeneration in which the muscle was pale, soft, and friable; microscopic examination showed accumulation of fatty droplets within the sarcolemma. Quain[4] was the first to recognize that the latter condition was associated with obstruction of the nutrient coronary artery branch. In a 1968 analysis of Quain's cases, Morgan[5] concluded that most were examples of ischemic heart disease, some with acute infarction. However, Gallavardin,[6] in 1900, recognized that the diffuse process found only on microscopic examination also accompanied cachectic, anoxemic, and anemic states. Thus, most of the attention to the fatty heart in the 19th century related to degenerative changes secondary to coronary disease or other conditions such as severe anemia and cachexia.

However, a possible relation between obesity, the heart, and sudden death was postulated in 1806 by Corvisart,[7] who described adipose tissue surrounding the heart; he suggested that in obese people the heart was oppressed by enveloping fat, which sometimes caused sudden death. In 1847 William Harvey[8,9] dissected the body of a corpulent man named Thomas Parr and found that "the heart was large, thick and fibrous, with a considerable quantity of adhering fat, both in its circum-

From: Alpert MA, and Alexander JK, (eds). *The Heart and Lung in Obesity.* Armonk, NY: Futura Publishing Company, Inc., © 1998.

ference and over its septum." Harvey states, "shortly before his death I had observed that his face was livid, he suffered from difficult breathing and orthopnea." Thus, in retrospect, this may have been the first observation of the cardiomyopathy of obesity. A propensity to sudden death with obesity had been previously noted by Celsus[10] (aphorism no. 11) and Hippocrates[11] in his often quoted aphorism no. 44, "Sudden death is more common in those that are naturally fat than in the lean."

Despite the considerable interest in the "fatty heart" for over a century, it was not until 1933 with the publication *Adiposity of the Heart* by Smith and Willius that the relation between obesity and heart weight was described, and the association of severe obesity with congestive heart failure (CHF) was appreciated.[12] Having previously established a relation between heart weight and body weight,[13] the authors recorded cardiac findings at autopsy in 135 patients with an average excess weight of 60% (20.5 kg), ranging from 14% (9.5 kg) to 170% (157.3 kg). The authors found that in almost all the obese subjects, the heart weight was greater than that predicted at normal body weight. In nine normotensive subjects with varying degrees of cardiac failure on clinical grounds, no evidence of primary cardiac disease was found at necropsy. Four of these, all extremely obese, had autopsy evidence of CHF and three died of heart failure. One of those who died of heart failure was a 33-year-old man with a body weight of 250 kg and a heart weight of 929 g. Although the authors ascribed the increased heart weight to excess epicardial fat, a concept that was later challenged, this was the first documentation in recent times of heart failure associated with obesity. Subsequently, in 1939 a case report from the Mayo Clinic,[14] coauthored by Willius, recorded heart failure in a 51-year-old man weighing 137 kg. The patient was cyanotic, had elevated blood volume, and polycythemia. The authors' diagnosis was pulmonary hypertension and cor pulmonale in view of right axis deviation in the electrocardiogram. After this report, nothing further appeared on the subject, at least in American literature, for the next 16 years. In 1955, Auchincloss et al[15] published an abstract "Polycythemia of Unknown Cause with Alveolar Hypoventilation," which reported heart failure in a young man with marked obesity, pulmonary hypertension (95/50 mm Hg), and a high cardiac output. This was the beginning of an era of renewed interest in the cardiopulmonary effects of obesity, with several case reports to follow in 1956 of heart failure with extreme obesity. Three patients with heart failure were reported by Estes et al,[16] and two other reports with autopsy findings in two patients who died of heart failure followed shortly thereafter.[17, 18] Interest at that time was further kindled by the paper of Burwell et al[19] describing Pickwickian syndrome[19] in a very obese patient.

Clinical features of Pickwickian syndrome, as defined by the authors, appear in Table 1. The term Pickwickian was derived from the description of somnolent fat boy Joe by Charles Dickens in the *Pickwick Papers*.[20] Although something of a misnomer[21] because somnolence was the only feature of the syndrome that character had, it was destined to become a familiar term in medical literature. The cardiac component was thought to be failure of the RV because hypoxemia and hypercapnia would foster pulmonary hypertension, and the finding of a normal pulmonary wedge pressure with pulmonary hypertension in similar patients had been previously reported by Sieker et al[22] in abstract form. This observation was derived from a single patient with mean pulmonary artery pressure of 25 mm Hg and a pulmonary wedge pressure of 3 mm Hg in a subsequent report by the same group.[16] Thus, it came about that marked obesity was designated as a cause of cor pulmonale in textbooks of medicine for more than 10 years thereafter. This concept was immediately accepted because of the diagnosis of heart failure due to cor pulmonale in reports with autopsy findings of RV hypertrophy in two cases of marked obesity appearing the same year[17,18] and in two other cases the following year.[23,24] However, this was not completely without exception. In 1957, Lillington et al[25] reported bilateral ventricular hypertrophy and pulmonary congestion at necropsy in an extremely obese man who died of massive pulmonary embolism, as well as reporting pulmonary congestion in other extremely obese subjects. These authors were the first to raise the question of left-sided cardiac involvement with obesity, stating, "the possible presence and importance of left cardiac failure cannot be summarily dismissed." Nevertheless, the assumption that cor pulmonale characterized heart failure secondary to extreme obesity remained predominant.

In 1959, Alexander and Dennis[26] reported that right heart catheterization of 40 extremely obese patients had demonstrated pulmonary hy-

---

Table 1
Clinical Features of the Pickwickian Syndrome

1. Obesity, marked
2. Somnolence
3. Twitching
4. Cyanosis
5. Periodic respiration
6. Polycythemia, secondary
7. Right ventricular hypertrophy
8. Right ventricular failure

---

pertension at rest or during exercise in the majority, and that it was accompanied by elevation of pulmonary wedge pressure, which suggested elevation of left ventricular (LV) filling pressure as the underlying mechanism. In 1962, it was pointed out by Alexander et al[27] that in the autopsy studies of extremely obese subjects previously cited as cases of cor pulmonale,[17,18,22,23] LV hypertrophy and pulmonary congestion had been present in each instance. Thus, the concept of cor pulmonale as the sole mechanism of heart failure with extreme obesity, even in the setting of hypoventilation, was seriously challenged. It was not until 1965 when a more critical appraisal of cardiac findings at necropsy by Amad et al in patients with long-standing severe obesity appeared; this reconfirmed the increase in heart weight observed by Smith and Willius,[12] but demonstrated that it was largely secondary to LV hypertrophy.[28] Of 12 patients examined, LV wall thickness was increased in all 11 where noted, and one patient had increase in RV thickness as well. Three of these patients died of heart failure with severe pulmonary and visceral congestion. Microscopic examination of the LV revealed myocyte hypertrophy in all cases. These pathological findings and the earlier hemodynamic studies established a basis for CHF in extreme obesity without other cause, increased heart weight secondary to LV hypertrophy rather than increased epicardial fat, and lack of evidence to support the concept of cor pulmonale as the sole mechanism of failure. Later case reports[29–31] and pathological studies of a series of extremely obese subjects[32,33] reconfirmed these observations. Morbid obesity is no longer listed as a cause of cor pulmonale, although increased pulmonary vascular resistance may be superimposed on underlying LV dysfunction in those subjects with hypoventilation.[34] Similarly, use of the engaging term Pickwickian syndrome, in vogue for over 25 years, has been abandoned in favor of "hypoventilation syndrome of obesity." This is probably just as well because it was a misnomer to begin with and the feature of cor pulmonale in its definition has proved to be a misconception.

A few years after recognizing that morbid obesity might lead to CHF, hemodynamic studies in these subjects first appeared.[35] With marked obesity, significant increments in plasma and total blood volume were found, which explained an increase in the size of the vascular bed. The increase in blood volume was paralleled by an increase in cardiac output, both of which correlated with the amount of excess body over the ideal body weight. Active metabolism of adipose tissue increased body oxygen consumption and correlated with body weight.[36] A large proportion of the high cardiac output in obese subjects supplied adipose tissue.[35] Similar findings were later extended to include very obese hypertensive patients.[37] Pulmonary hypertension with an accompanying rise in pulmonary wedge pressure at rest or during exercise was reported.[38] These characteristics were later confirmed[39, 40] also with observations of elevated LV filling pressure[41,42] and diminished LV chamber compliance.[42,43] Partial reversibility of these hemodynamic changes after weight reduction was later documented.[41,44]

A study by Kasper et al[45] of obese patients with CHF showed a high cardiac output as compared with other patients with dilated cardiomyopathy, as well as absence of microscopic changes other than myocyte hypertrophy on endocardial biopsy.

With the application of echocardiographic and radionuclide methodology, further appraisal of anatomical and functional features of obesity cardiomyopathy followed. In what appears to be the first echocardiographic study in morbidly obese subjects two functional patterns were observed by Alexander et al.[43] In one group, there was a normal or quasi-normal ejection fraction and normal ratio of LV wall thickness to chamber radius, indicating a normal wall stress. In the second group, LV end-diastolic volume was significantly increased, with an abnormal ratio of wall thickness to chamber radius, compatible with elevated LV wall stress. In this latter group, reduction in ejection fraction and mean circumferential fiber shortening rate indicated LV systolic dysfunction. It was postulated that all obese cardiomyopathic patients were subject to LV diastolic dysfunction and some to systolic dysfunction secondary to "inadequate" hypertrophy. Echocardiographic estimates of increased LV mass in extremely obese subjects with or without hypertension confirmed the LV hypertrophy found in earlier pathological studies,[46] and eccentric hypertrophy was documented in obese hypertensive patients.[47] In 1985, Nakajima et al[48] first called attention to the importance of obesity duration in relation to echocardiographic findings. In moderately obese subjects, duration of obesity correlated positively with LV dimension, radius to wall thickness ratio, and stroke index. LV wall thickness, end-systolic wall stress, and calculated cardiac output were significantly higher in those with obesity of more than 15 years' duration as compared with those with obesity of shorter duration. These observations were subsequently extended by Alpert et al[49] in morbidly obese subjects to include decrements in LV fractional shortening (LVFS) and filling velocity over time.

Increase in LV mass was found to parallel body mass index (BMI) over a wide range in the 1991 Framingham Heart Study report.[50] Attention to diastolic LV function in obesity soon developed. In 1989, Egan et al[51] had found that relative weight was the single best predictor of peak LV filling rate as assessed by radionuclide ventriculography in mild hypertensives. In 1991, the first Doppler study of LV filling velocity with moderately severe obesity (BMI $31 \pm$ kg/m^2) by Grossman et al[52] indicated that peak LV filling velocity was reduced and correlated negatively with LV mass and BMI.[52] Doppler studies of LV filling in morbidly obese subjects, reported by Zarich et al[53] in 1991, further confirmed the presence of LV diastolic dysfunction by demonstrating diminished filling velocities and increased atrial contribution to stroke velocity.

Later studies by Alpert et al[54] in morbid obesity confirmed the relation between impairment of LV filling and increasing ventricular mass, and emphasized the importance of loading conditions.

Although hemodynamic alterations after weight loss in very obese subjects had been reported in the 1970s, it was not until 1985 in a study by Alpert et al[55] that the effect of weight loss on cardiac morphology and LV function was explored. In morbidly obese subjects, reduction in mean blood pressure was accompanied by diminution in LV dimension when enlarged preoperatively, and improvement in LVFS when reduced preoperatively. Subsequently, in a study of 12 morbidly obese subjects losing 55 kg (mean) after gastroplasty, Alaud-din et al[56] reported, by radionuclide angiography, improvement in ejection fraction both at rest and during exercise. In recent years, several echocardiographic studies by Alpert and colleagues[57] have further clarified the effects of weight loss on cardiac anatomy and function in the morbidly obese. Improvement in LVFS is closely related to alterations in loading conditions, particularly reduced systolic blood pressure and end-systolic wall stress.[58] In those with an elevated LV mass/height index, reduction in ventricular mass and more favorable loading conditions with weight loss are accompanied by improvement in Doppler indices of LV filling such as E to A ratio and E wave deceleration time.[59] In normotensive and hypertensive subjects with moderately severe obesity, weight loss is accompanied by a reduction in LV mass.[60]

Thus, the evolution of our understanding of the cardiomyopathy of obesity has been very slow, although there has been some acceleration in recent years. It was almost 25 years before the pathological finding of heart failure in obese subjects without other apparent cause was recognized by Smith and Willius[12] in 1933 as a clinical entity, and another 10 years or so before it was appreciated that the condition was characterized by LV dysfunction. Another 20 years passed before the hemodynamic and ventricular functional aspects were reasonably well defined. The advent of bariatric surgery in combination with echocardiographic and radionuclide methodology has provided an opportunity to gain considerable insight into pathophysiological mechanisms in recent years. It is not clear that hemodynamic factors alone can account for the impressive LV hypertrophy that occurs with weight gain, nor the regression of hypertrophy with weight loss. It is not unreasonable to speculate that the same genetic factors predisposing to obesity may also impact upon LV mass. An interesting observation in this regard is by Sasson et al[61] who suggested that insulin resistance is an important independent contributing factor to LV mass in nondiabetic obese subjects. Clearly, further study at the molecular level is needed.

References

1. Bedford E: The study of fatty heart. A disease of Victorian times. *Br Heart J* 34:23–28, 1972.
2. Senac JB: *Traite'de la structure du coeur, de son action, et de ses maladies,* 2nd ed. Vol. 2. Mequignon, Paris, 1783, p. 384.
3. Laennec RTH: *De l'Auscultation Mediate ou Traite'du Diagnostic des Maladies des Poumons et du Coeur,* Vol. 2. Brosson and Chaudé, Paris, 1819, p.295.
4. Quain R: Fatty disease of the heart. *Medicosurg Transact* 33:121, 1985.
5. Morgan AD: Some forms of undiagnosed coronary disease in nineteenth century England. *Med Hist* 12:344, 1968.
6. Gallavardin L: *La Degenerescence Graisseuse du Myocarde.* J.B. Bailliere, Paris. 1900.
7. Corvisart JN: *Essai sur les Maladies et les Lesions Organiques du Coeur et des Gros Vaisseaux.* Migneret, Paris, 1806.
8. Harvey W: Anatomical examination of the body of Thomas Parr. In Harvey W (ed): *Works of William Harvey, translated from the Latin by Robert Willis.* Sydenham Society, London, 1847, p. 589.
9. Ford WJ: Old Parr. *Bull Hist Med* 24:219–226, 1950.
10. Sprengell CJ: *The aphorisms of Hippocrates and the sentences of Celsus.* K. Bonwick, et al. London, 1708.
11. Chadwick J, Mann WN: *The Medical Works of Hippocrates. Aphorisms,* Sect. II, 44. Charles C. Thomas, Springfield, IL, 1950, p. 154.
12. Smith HL, Willius FA: Adiposity of the heart. *Arch Intern Med* 52:911–931, 1933.
13. Smith HL: The relation of the weight of the heart to the weight of the body, and of the weight of the heart to age. *Am Heart J* 4:79–93, 1928.
14. Olsen AM, Willius FA: Clinic on cardiac failure resulting from pulmonary hypertension (Ayerza's Disease) complicated by arterial hypertension and marked obesity. *Proc Staff Meetings Mayo Clinic* 14:89–91, 1939.
15. Auchincloss JH Jr, Cook E, Renzetti A: Polycythemia of unknown cause with alveolar hypoventilation. *Clin Res Proc* 3:31–32, 1955.
16. Ester EH Jr, Sieker HO, McIntosh HD, et al: Reversible cardiopulmonary syndrome with extreme obesity. *Circulation* 16:179–187, 1957.
17. Counihan TB: Heart failure due to extreme obesity. *Br Heart J* 38:425–426, 1956.
18. Carroll D: A peculiar type of cardiopulmonary failure associated with obesity. *Am J Med* 21:819–824, 1956.
19. Burwell CS, Robin ED, Whaley RD, et al: Extreme obesity associated with hypoventilation—a Pickwickian syndrome. *Am J Med* 21:811–818, 1956.
20. Dickens C: The Posthumous Papers of the Pickwick Club. Chapman and Hall, London 1837.

21. Berlyne GM: The cardiorespiratory syndrome of extreme obesity. *Lancet* 2:939–930, 1958.
22. Sieker HO, Estes EH Jr, Kelser GA, et al: A cardiopulmonary syndrome associated with extreme obesity. *J Clin Invest* 34:916, 1955.
23. Seide MJ: Heart failure due to extreme obesity. *N Engl J Med* 257: 1227–1230, 1957.
24. Soriano AQ, Durham JR Jr: Pickwickian syndrome. *Del State Med J* 29: 153–154, 1957.
25. Lillington GA, Anderson MA, Brandenberg RO: The cardiorespiratory syndrome of obesity. *Dis Chest* 32:1–20, 1957.
26. Alexander JK, Dennis EW: Circulatory dynamics in extreme obesity. *Circulation* 20:662, 1959.
27. Alexander JK, Amad KH, Cole VW: Observations on some clinical features of extreme obesity with particular reference to cardiorespiratory effects. *Am J Med* 32:512–524, 1962.
28. Amad KH, Brennan JC, Alexander JK: The cardiac pathology of obesity. *Circulation* 32:740–745, 1965.
29. MacGregor MI, Block AJ, Ball WC Jr: Serious complications and sudden death in Pickwickian syndrome. *Johns Hopkins Med J* 126:279–295, 1970.
30. James TN, Frame B, Coates EO: De subitaneis mortibus III: Pickwickian syndrome. *Circulation* 48:1311–1320, 1973.
31. Massive obesity and cardiac failure. Barnes Hospital Clinopathologic Conference. *Am J Med* 64:827–833, 1978.
32. Alexander JK, Pettigrove JK: Obesity and congestive heart failure. *Geriatrics* 22:101–108, 1967.
33. Warnes CA, Roberts WC: The heart in massive (more than 300 pounds or 136 kilograms) obesity: Analysis of 12 patients studied at necropsy. *Am J Cardiol* 54:1087–1091, 1984.
34. Kaltman AJ, Goldring RM: Role of circulatory congestion in the cardiorespiratory failure of obesity. *Am J Med* 60:645–653, 1976.
35. Alexander JK, Dennis EW, Smith WG, et al: Blood volume, cardiac output and distribution of systemic blood flow in extreme obesity. *Cardiovasc Res Center Bull* 1:39–44, 1962.
36. White RE, Alexander JK: Body oxygen consumption and pulmonary ventilation in obese subjects. *J Appl Physiol* 20: 197–201, 1965.
37. Messerli FH, Christie B, DeCarvallo JGR, et al: Obesity and essential hypertension. Hemodynamics, intravascular volume, sodium excretion and plasma renin activity. *Arch Intern Med* 141:81–85, 1981.
38. Alexander JK: Obesity and the circulation. *Mod Concepts Cardiovasc Dis* 32:799–803, 1963.
39. Bachman L, Freyschuss U, Hallberg D, et al: Cardiovascular function in extreme obesity. *Acta Med Scand* 193:799–803, 1963.
40. Agarwal N, Shibutani R, Sanfilippo JA, et al: Hemodynamic and respiratory changes in surgery of the morbidly obese. *Surgery* 92:226–234, 1982.
41. Alexander JK, Peterson KL: Cardiovascular effects of weight reduction. *Circulation* 45:310–318, 1972.
42. Di Devitiis O, Fazio S, Petitto M, et al: Obesity and cardiac function. *Circulation* 64:477–482, 1981.
43. Alexander JK, Woodard CB, Quinones MA, et al: Heart failure from obe-

sity. In Mancini M, Lewis B, Contaldo F (eds): *Medical Complications of Obesity.* Academic Press, London, 1978, pp. 179–187.

44. Backman L, Freyschuss U, Hallberg D, et al: Reversibility of cardiovascular changes in extreme obesity. *Acta Med Scand* 205:367–373, 1979.
45. Kasper EK, Hruban RH, Baughman KL: Cardiomyopathy of obesity: A clinicopathologic evaluation of 43 obese patients with heart failure. *Am J Cardiol* 70:921–924, 1992.
46. Cueto Garcia L, Laredo C, Arriaga J, et al: Echocardiographic findings in obesity. *Rev Invest Clin* 34:235–241, 1982.
47. Messerli FH, Sundgaard-Riise K, Reisin ED, et al: Dimorphic cardiac adaptation to obesity and arterial hypertension. *Ann Intern Med* 99:757–761, 1983
48. Nakajima T, Jujioka S, Tokunaga K, et al: Non-invasive study of left ventricular performance in obese patients: Influence of duration of obesity. *Circulation* 71:481–486, 1985.
49. Alpert MA, Lambert CR, Panayiotou H, et al: Relation of duration of obesity to left ventricular mass, systolic function and diastolic filling, and effect of weight loss. *Am J Cardiol* 76:1194–1197, 1995.
50. Lauer MS, Anderson KM, Kannel WB, et al: The impact of obesity on left ventricular mass and geometry: The Framingham Heart Study. *JAMA* 266:231–236, 1991.
51. Egan B, Fitzpatrick A, Juni J, et al: Importance of overweight in studies of left ventricular hypertrophy and diastolic function in mild systemic hypertension. *Am J Cardiol* 64:752–755, 1989.
52. Grossman E, Oren S, Messerli FH: Left ventricular filling in the systemic hypertension of obesity. *Am J Cardiol* 68:57–60, 1991.
53. Zarich SW, Kowalchuk GJ, McGuire MP, et al: Left ventricular abnormalities in asymptomatic morbid obesity. *Am J Cardiol* 68:377–381, 1991.
54. Alpert MA, Lambert CR, Terry BE, et al: Influence of left ventricular mass on left ventricular diastolic filling in normotensive morbid obesity. *Am Heart J* 130:1068–1073, 1995.
55. Alpert MA, Terry BE, Kelly DL: Effect of weight loss on cardiac chamber size, wall thickness and left ventricular function in patients who were morbidly obese. *Am J Cardiol* 55:783–786, 1985.
56. Alaud-din A, Meterissian S, Lisbona R, et al: Assessment of cardiac function in patients who were morbidly obese. *Surgery* 108:809–818, 1990.
57. Alpert MA, Lambert CR, Terry BE, et al: Effect of weight loss on left ventricular mass in non-hypertensive morbidly obese patients. *Am J Cardiol* 73:918–921, 1994
58. Alpert MA, Terry BE, Lambert CR, et al: Factors influencing left ventricular systolic function in non-hypertensive morbidly obese patients, and effect of weight loss induced by gastroplasty. *Am J Cardiol* 71:733–737, 1993.
59. Alpert MA, Lambert CR, Terry BE, et al: Effect of weight loss on left ventricular diastolic filling in morbid obesity. *Am J Cardiol* 76:1198–1201, 1995.
60. Himeno E, Nishino K, Nakashima Y, et al: Weight reduction regresses left ventricular mass regardless of blood pressure level in obese subjects. *Am Heart J* 131:313–319, 1996.
61. Sasson Z, Rasooly Y, Bhesania T, et al: Insulin resistance is an important determinant of left ventricular mass in the obese. *Circulation* 88:1431–1436, 1993.

Chapter 2

Effect of Obesity on Myocardial Metabolism, Morphology, and Function in the Obese (fa/fa) Zucker Rat

Stephen W. Schaffer, PhD

Introduction

A number of rodent models have been developed to study the complex interplay between obesity, hyperinsulinemia, and glucose intolerance. The most widely studied animal models of obesity are the Zucker (fa/fa) obese rat, the obese (ob/ob) mouse, and the CBL/57 strain (db/db) mouse.[1–3] Although these animal models share many metabolic characteristics, the two mouse strains are genetically predisposed to develop noninsulin-dependent diabetes, while the Zucker (fa/fa) rat only exhibits moderate basal hyperglycemia and is considered by most investigators a more appropriate model of obesity. Two other genetic strains of obese rats have been developed that show promise as models of obesity in combination with some other cardiovascular complication. The obese SHR rat resembles the newly described clinical condition, syndrome X, which is characterized by hypertriglyceridemia, hypertension, hyperglycemia, and hyperinsulinemia,[4] while the recently developed JCR:LA-cp rat has attracted considerable attention because it is the only strain of obese rats to develop atherosclerosis.[5]

From: Alpert MA, and Alexander JK, (eds). *The Heart and Lung in Obesity.* Armonk, NY: Futura Publishing Company, Inc., © 1998.

The genetically obese Zucker (fa/fa) rat has an autosomal recessive mutation on chromosome 5, which is referred to as the *fa* gene.[6] Homozygotes with this abnormal gene are indistinguishable from nonobese littermates until the third or fourth week of age. By 5 weeks of age, the obese rat shows a significant increase in body weight and percent body lipid content.[3] The percent body lipid content continues to increase until about week 14, at which time the rat continues to gain body weight without a change in percent body lipid.[7] Upon reaching adulthood, nearly 50% of the rat's body weight is lipid, which is five times the normal.

Because obesity is a complex disorder, it is not surprising that the cause of lipid accumulation in the Zucker (fa/fa) rat is inadequately understood. One of the earliest abnormalities described in the obese rat is an increase on plasma triglyceride levels.[8] This is related in part to an elevation in lipogenesis, fatty acid esterification, and very low-density lipoprotein production by the liver.[3, 9] The obese rat also consumes more food than lean control rats, therefore, diet also is an important source of elevated plasma triglyceride content. The increase in plasma lipid levels, combined with elevated lipoprotein lipase activity, ensure a ready supply of fatty acids for the adipocyte of the Zucker rat.[3, 10–12] Moderate increases in fat storage occur as early as 1 week of age, well before the development of other metabolic defects. After weaning, the obese rat becomes hyperinsulinemic and a burst of fat storage occurs.[13] Ultimately, the obese Zucker rat exhibits a dramatic increase in both adipocyte size and number.[3]

Myocardial Energy Metabolism in the Obese Zucker Rat

Over 90% of the adenosine triphosphate (ATP) required for maintenance of normal myocardial contractile function is derived from the metabolism of glucose and fatty acids. In the well-oxygenated heart, fatty acids are utilized in preference to glucose. However, glucose becomes an important substrate postprandially and at high levels of cardiac work.[14] Because the myocardium is an aerobic tissue, most of the ATP generated from glucose metabolism is derived from glucose oxidation rather than anaerobic metabolism.

The metabolism of fatty acids by the heart also depends on aerobic metabolism. The main source of fatty acids for the heart is albumin-bound free fatty acids and fatty acids supplied by plasma lipoproteins, both of which are elevated in the obese Zucker rat.[3, 12] Because fatty acid uptake is linearly dependent on plasma free fatty acid content (Figure 1), delivery of fatty acids to the heart is elevated in the obese Zucker rat.[14]

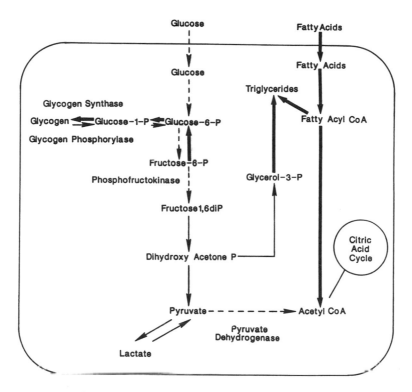

Figure 1. Effect of obesity on myocardial glucose and fatty acid metabolism. Blood fatty acid levels of the obese Zucker rat are elevated, causing fatty acid uptake by the heart to rise. The increased availability of fatty acid substrate results in enhanced rated of both β-oxidation and triglyceride synthesis. In accordance with the known competition between fatty acids and glucose as energy sources, myocardial glucose metabolism is severely impaired in the obese Zucker rat. Two key steps in the metabolism of glucose are inhibited; phosphofructokinase, and pyruvate dehydrogenase. The inhibition of phosphofructokinase serves as a bottleneck, which prevents adequate flux of substrate through the glycolytic pathway. Instead, substrate is diverted into glycogen synthesis. **Bold** and **dashed** arrows represent obesity-induced increases and decreases, respectively, in flux through individual steps in a metabolic pathway

Once the fatty acids enter the heart, they become associated with fatty acid binding proteins, which target them to one of the pathways of fatty acid metabolism. In the well-oxygenated heart, most of the fatty acid pool undergoes β-oxidation; however, significant elevations in tissue fatty acid content increases the proportion of lipids diverted to triglyceride synthesis (Figure 1). Thus, it is not surprising that in the heart of the obese Zucker rat triglyceride levels increase more than twofold.[15]

The triglyceride pool is an important endogenous source of fatty acids that can be utilized if circulating fatty acid levels are reduced.[14] Rösen et al[16] have shown that the myocardial endogenous triglyceride pool of the obese Zucker rat can provide up to 80% to 90% of the heart's energy needs. Interestingly, the extent of endogenous fatty acid mobilization is an important feature distinguishing the metabolic properties of the obese Zucker rat from those of its lean littermates. Hearts of the lean Zucker rats perfused with buffer containing glucose (plus insulin) as the sole exogenous substrate rely on endogenous fatty acid metabolism for only 25% of its adenosine triphosphate (ATP) needs. By contrast, under identical perfusion conditions, more than 80% of ATP generated by the heart of the obese Zucker rat is obtained from β-oxidation.[16]

The rate of both exogenous and endogenous fatty acid metabolism is partially limited by the extent of flux through the β-oxidation and citric acid cycle pathways.[14] Several factors regulate β-oxidation flux, including tissue levels of carnitine and coenzyme A (CoA), the rate of oxidative phosphorylation (ie, the mitochondrial $NADH/NAD^+$ ratio), the shunting of acetyl CoA into the citric acid cycle (ie, the mitochondrial acetyl CoA/CoA ratio), and the presence of malonyl CoA in the cytosol.[17,18] Although limited information is available on the status of these regulatory factors in the heart of the obese Zucker rat, studies examining fatty acid oxidation in the isolated heart suggest that fatty acid availability, rather than the rate of β-oxidation, determines the contribution of fatty acid metabolism to overall ATP generation in the heart of the obese Zucker rat.[16] This conclusion is based on the assumption that the rate of fatty acid oxidation is equal to the portion of oxygen consumption not due to glucose oxidation. Although this assumption is scientifically sound in the normal rat, it may not be valid in the pathological state of obesity. This latter view is held by Quignard-Boulange et al,[19] who found that β-oxidation of exogenous oleate is depressed in neonatal myocytes from obese Zucker rats compared to lean controls. Because both the incorporation of ^{14}C-oleate into neutral lipids and the rate of glucose oxidation are also diminished in the abnormal neonatal myocyte, Quignard-Boulange et al[19] have concluded that a defect in the entire metabolic machinery exists in heart cells of the obese Zucker rat. While it is possible that obesity could induce multiple metabolic defects, a more probable explanation for the broad decline in cellular energy metabolism is a reduction in ATP demand. The most dominant predictor of ATP demand in the myocyte is contractile function, therefore, a change in contractile function could account for the abnormal metabolic flux pattern of the obese Zucker rat. Unfortunately, the contractile status of the neonatal myocyte of the obese Zucker rat has not been examined.

While there is some debate regarding the cause of altered fatty acid metabolism in the heart of the obese Zucker rat, there is general agreement regarding the impairment in glucose metabolism. According to the classic studies of Randle and coworkers,[20] enhanced fatty acid oxidation leads to a cellular increase in the level of two metabolic products, citrate and acetyl-coenzyme A (AcCoA), which are potent inhibitors of rate-limiting steps in glucose metabolism. Citrate, an effective inhibitor of the glycolytic enzyme phosphofructokinase, is elevated in the heart of the obese Zucker rat.[16] Consequently, basal, as well as epinephrine-mediated activation of phosphofructokinase, is severely impaired in the heart of the obese rat.[21] The other important metabolic end product of fatty acid oxidation, AcCoA, inhibits pyruvate dehydrogenase activity. Although the activity of pyruvate dehydrogenase in the heart of the obese Zucker rat has never been directly evaluated, flux measurements suggest that the enzyme exists in a partially inhibited state.[16] Both enzymes have profound effects on glucose metabolism, with impaired phosphofructokinase severely slowing glycolytic flux and diminished pyruvate dehydrogenase activity reducing the flow of triose units into the citric acid cycle. Thus, both anaerobic ATP generation and the oxidation of triose units by citric acid cycle are severely diminished in the heart of the obese Zucker rat (Figure 1).

Obesity-mediated reductions in glycolytic flux also affect glycogen metabolism. Since phosphofructokinase is severely inhibited in the heart of the obese rat, glucose is diverted into glycogen synthesis (Figure 1). Thus, while hearts of the lean Zucker rat experience a significant rate of glycogenolysis, glycogen levels are well preserved in the heart of the obese rat.[16]

Despite its overreliance on fatty acid metabolism for ATP generation, the heart of the obese Zucker rat is not energy compromised; all measurements of high energy phosphate status, including energy charge, fall within normal range.[16] Moreover, the rate of myocardial ATP generation is compatible in the lean and obese Zucker rat.

Impaired Insulin Responsiveness in the Myocardium of the Obese Zucker Rat

A tightly regulated feedback loop exists between plasma glucose levels and plasma insulin content of the lean Zucker rat (Figure 2). This regulation is illustrated by the characteristic response to a standard glucose tolerance test.[7,12] After a glucose challenge, plasma insulin levels rise, causing enhanced glucose uptake by peripheral tissues and suppression

A. Feedback Loop in Lean Zucker Rat

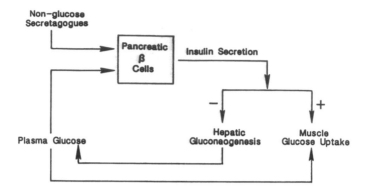

B. Feedback Loop in Obese Zucker Rat

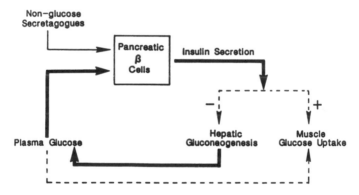

Figure 2. Normal feedback loop for insulin and glucose. **Top:** Pancreatic insulin production secretion is regulated by plasma levels of glucose and nonglucose secretagogues. Once secreted, insulin acts to inhibit glucose synthesis by the liver and stimulate glucose uptake by muscle. This regulation of hepatic glucose production and peripheral glucose utilization maintains blood glucose levels within the normal range. When blood glucose content rises, insulin secretion is enhanced, which reduces hepatic gluconeogenesis and stimulated muscle glucose uptake, rapidly restoring a balance between plasma glucose and insulin levels. **Bottom:** Operation of the feedback loop in the insulin-resistant, obese Zucker rate. The liver and muscle of the obese Zucker rat exhibits severe insulin resistance. Thus, normal blood insulin levels are unable to adequately regulate hepatic gluconeogenesis and myocoyte glucose utilization. Consequently, plasma glucose levels increase. This in turn acts to elevate the rate of insulin secretion by the pancreatic β-cells. Blood insulin levels rise and partially overcome the defect at the level of the liver and muscle. A new steady state is established, characterized by severe hyperinsulinemia and mild hyperglycemia. **Bold** and **dashed arrows** represent obesity-induced increases and decreases, respectively, in steps of the glucose-insulin feedback loop.

of glucose production by the liver.[22] Consequently, plasma glucose levels rapidly return to resting levels. Lower glucose levels in turn reduce the rate of pancreatic insulin secretion and plasma insulin levels fall.

The response of the 15-week-old obese Zucker rat to a glucose challenge is very different from that of the lean control (Figure 2). After a glucose challenge, plasma glucose and insulin increase to peak levels, which are significantly greater than those observed in the lean control rat.[12] This condition of hyperinsulinemia and hyperglycemia also occurs in noninsulin-dependent diabetes and has been attributed to the severe insulin resistant state of the animal.[22] In the 15-week-old obese Zucker rat, peripheral insulin resistance is fairly severe and has been shown to interfere with the regulation of hepatic gluconeogenesis and insulin-stimulated glucose transport.[16, 23] Consequently, plasma glucose levels rise inordinately, which in turn triggers further pancreatic insulin secretion. The extra insulin partially overcomes the state of insulin resistance and glucose levels begin to fall. Ultimately, a new steady state is established, in which the animal exhibits severe hyperinsulinemia and mild hyperglycemia. This state of glucose intolerance and insulin resistance is most severe in the 15-week-old obese Zucker rat.[7] Younger obese rats (2 to 5 weeks of age) exhibit hyperinsulinemia, but are glucose tolerant, while older obese rats (50 weeks of age) are characterized by only moderate elevations in serum insulin levels.

Glucose transport by the heart is an insulin-responsive process; therefore, it is not surprising that insulin-mediated enhancement of myocardial glucose transport is impaired in the insulin resistant, obese Zucker rat.[16, 24, 25] The biochemical mechanism underlying this defect has been an area of considerable interest and speculation. Uphues et al[26] have attributed the defect to a series of biochemical abnormalities, including reduced myocardial expression of the GLUT 4 glucose transport, lower GLUT 4 levels in the microsomal membrane fraction, and defective recruitment of GLUT 4 to the plasma membrane in response to insulin. Although Zaninetti et al[25] have also reported a reduction in the number of glucose transporters translocated to the plasma membrane in response to insulin, they have provided evidence that the activity of the translocated transported is also reduced. This idea is further supported by the observation that contractile-induced activation of glucose transport is also defective in the hearts of obese rats.[25]

While most studies have focused on the biochemistry of glucose transporter activation, a few studies have examined earlier steps in the insulin signal transduction pathway. Slieker et al[27] have reported that insulin receptor tyrosine kinase activity is severely depressed in hind limb skeletal muscle of the obese Zucker rat. Although this initial phosphorylation step has not been studied in the heart of the obese Zucker rat, the fact that the insulin-mediated positive inotropic effect is seemingly normal in the heart of the obese Zucker rat implies that the early steps in the signal transduction pathway of insulin must be operating normally.[16] However, Van de Werve et al[28] have argued that a later step in the insulin signaling cascade, namely protein kinase C activation, is abnormal. They found that "restoration" of protein kinase C activity by treatment of the isolated heart with the calcium ionophore A23187, largely restores insulin-mediated stimulation of glucose transport. Moreover, downregulation of protein kinase C through daily administration of phorbol myristate acetate produces an insulin-resistant condition resembling that observed in the obese rat.[28]

Cardiac Structure and Hemodynamic Alterations in the Obese Zucker Rat

Cardiac hypertrophy is an important feature of obesity in both man and animals.[29,30] In the absence of other cardiovascular complications, human obesity leads to eccentric hypertrophy (caused by volume overload). By contrast, mixed eccentric and concentric hypertrophy predominates in obese individuals with coexisting hypertension. Despite its pathological importance, only one study has examined the type of hypertrophy that develops in the obese Zucker rat. In that study, the experimental group was mildly hypertensive and their hearts exhibited increases in both intraventricular volume and the ratio of wall thickness/internal radius.[30] These heart dimensions are characteristic of a mixed type of hypertrophy caused by a combination of pressure and volume overload. Yet, many colonies of obese Zucker rats are normotensive. Although heart structure has not been examined in the normotensive, obese rat based on clinical studies, it is logical to assume that the heart of these animals should be dilated as a result of volume overloading. More studies are required to confirm this hypothesis.

Age has a dramatic effect on the metabolic state of the obese Zucker rat; therefore, it is not surprising that age also affects the mechanical properties of the heart. In most studies, left ventricular pressure and the rate of pressure rise (dP/dt) are elevated in isolated hearts obtained from male obese rats younger than 19 weeks of age.[16,31] Cardiac output is also elevated in this age group, although the increase appears to be linked to the degree of cardiac hypertrophy; normalizing the data for heart weight usually eliminates the difference in cardiac output.[31] In these younger, obese rats inhibition of carnitine palmitoyl transferase I activity significantly increases contractile function, suggesting a link between energy metabolism and cardiac performance in these rats.[16]

In contrast to the younger obese rat, older obese animals consistently exhibit impaired contractile function. Paulson and Tahiliani[32] have found that both cardiac output (independent of heart weight) and cardiac work are significantly reduced in hearts of 38- to 44-week-old obese rats perfused with buffer containing 0.4 mM palmitate and 5.5 mM glucose, and equilibrated with a 95% O_2 and 5% CO_2 gas mix. In a related study, Segal et al[31] reported depressed cardiac output in a 19-week-old male and obese Zucker rats perfused with buffer containing 11 mM glucose and equilibrated with gas containing 45% nitrogen, 50% O_2, and 5% CO_2. Despite major differences in medium substrate and oxygen composition, similar ventricular function curves were generated in the two studies. Thus, the age of the obese rat is a more important determinant of ventricular function than perfusion medium composition. This observation supports the notion that in contrast to the younger obese rat impaired ATP production is not the basis for the observed impairment in contractile function of the older obese rat.

The mechanism underlying the obesity-induced contractile defects has not been widely investigated. In one of the few studies of its kind in the obese Zucker rat, Morris et al[33] reported a reduction in the expression of V_1, the myosin adenosine triphospatase (ATPase) isoform with the highest activity. Similar changes in V_1 occur in the diabetic and hypothyroid heart and are thought to contribute to the cardiomyopathies that develop in those conditions.[34] Another attractive candidate for the observed decline in cardiac contractility is the impaired Ca^{2+} movement. Vernimmen et al[35] have observed suppressed slow action potentials characteristic of the inward Ca^{2+} current in the heart of a 12-week-old obese Zucker rat. Although not examined to date, two lines of evidence make it likely that sarcoplasmic reticular Ca^{2+} transport will also be defective in the heart of the obese rat. First, sarcoplasmic reticular Ca^{2+} transport is defective in aortic smooth muscle of the obese Zucker rat.[36] Second, hypothyroidism and hyperinsulinemia, which coexist with the obese condition, are associated with impaired myocardial sarcoplasmic reticular Ca^{2+} pump activity.[34] Nevertheless, evidence supporting the involvement of abnormal Ca^{2+} movement in the contractile defects of the obese Zucker rat is minimal, indicating the need for further investigation.

Response to Effectors of Cardiac Mechanical Function

The obese Zucker rat develops several endocrine disorders, including hyperinsulinemia, hypothyroidism, impaired pituitary function, decreased growth hormone levels, reduced prolactin content, and diminished glucagon secretion.[3,37,38] Only some of the myocardial consequences of these neurohumoral defects have been examined.

The neurohumoral system most widely studied in the heart of the obese Zucker rat has been the β-adrenergic system. A consistent finding has been that obese male Zucker rats (ages 12 to 45 weeks) exhibit impaired myocardial responsiveness to β-adrenergic agonists, such as isoproterenol.[39–41] Typical of these studies is the work of Robberecht et al,[40] who observed a reduction in the maximal inotropic response of isoproterenol in papillary muscle preparations obtained from 30-week-old obese Zucker rats. Studies designed to uncover the basis for the abnormal isoproterenol response have ruled out altered adenylate cyclase activity as the cause.[41] A decline in β-adrenergic receptor number has also been considered a likely candidate for reduced isoproterenol responsiveness. However, the observed reduction in receptor number may merely reflect a dilution of the receptor population by hypertrophy rather than a down regulation of the receptor.[42] According to a study by Stressheim et al,[41] the interaction between the β-adrenergic receptor and the G_s coupling protein is probably the most important contributor to abnormal β-adrenergic responsiveness in the obese heart (Figure 3). They have pointed out that since the activation of one adrenergic receptor serves as an amplifier to activate a number of G_s proteins, the coupling process is a very sensitive target to control the responsiveness of catecholamines. Thus, the observed defect in the activation of the G_s coupling protein by the β-adrenergic system in the heart of the obese Zucker rat provides a logical explanation for impaired β-adrenergic responsiveness.

Other effectors, whose signal transduction pathways also proceed through the G_s coupling protein, exhibit impaired responses in the obese Zucker rat. Activation of cardiac muscle adenylate cyclase by glucagon (3 μM) are attenuated in 21% and 77%, respectively, in 12-week-old obese Zucker rats in comparison to nonobese controls.[39] Aging potentiates the severity of the defect; by 45 weeks of age, maximal stimulation of adenylate cyclase by glucagon and secretin is depressed 42% and 91%, respectively. Vasoactive intestinal peptide responsiveness is also severely depressed in the older obese rats.[39]

In contrast to adenylate cyclase-linked effectors, Auclar et al[43] have shown that α-adrenergic agonists, which activate a signal trans-

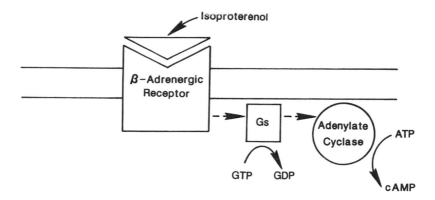

Figure 3. Effect of obesity on the signal transduction pathway of β-adrenergic system. The β-adrenergic agonist, isoproterenol, interacts with the β-adrenergic receptor, which in turn activated a G_s protein. The activated G_s protein stimulated adenylate cyclase to produce cAMP. In the heart of the obese Zucker rat, the activation of the G_s protein by occupied β-adrenergic receptor is impaired. Consequently, the stimulation of adenyate cyclase by β-adrenergic agonists is attenuated. The **dashed arrows** represent impaired coupling and activation of the step in the signal transduction pathway.

duction pathway leading to the stimulation of phospholipase C, appear to respond normally in the obese Zucker rat. Yet, because the study by Auclar et al[43] was restricted to an investigation of α-agonist-induced contractile and electrophysiological changes in young obese Zucker rats, further studies seem warranted. One important parameter not examined to date is the effect of obesity on α-adrenergic-induced myocyte growth. Also of keen interest is the involvement of other growth factors and regulators in the development of obesity-induced myocardial hypertrophy.

Summary

The Zucker rat (fa/fa) has been a useful model to ascertain the cardiovascular effects of obesity. These effects are age dependent, largely because the metabolic changes in the rat are also age dependent. The obese rat begins to gain weight by 5 weeks of age, at which point myocardial metabolism begins to favor the utilization of fatty acids. By the age of 15 weeks the animal is severely obese, his plasma glucose levels are mildly elevated, and his plasma insulin levels are dramatically increased. At this age, the heart exhibits characteristics of severe insulin resistance, including impaired basal and insulin-stimulated glucose metabolism: 80% to 90% of the heart's energy needs are derived from fatty acid metabolism. Myocardial mechanical function is enhanced in these animals, an effect related in part to the increase in cardiac size. By the time the animal reaches an age of 35 weeks, cardiac function has been severely compromised. The decrease in mechanical function is associated with the development of either eccentric hypertrophy (volume overload induced) or mixed hypertrophy (caused by volume and pressure overload). Although the hypertrophic cardiomyopathy that evolves has been partially characterized, little information is available regarding the mechanism underlying the development of this condition. Clearly, further studies providing insight into the causes of the cardiomyopathy are warranted.

References

1. Dubuc PU, Cahn PJ, Willis P: The effect of exercise and food restriction on obesity and diabetes in young ob/ob mice. *Int J Obes* 8:271–278, 1984.
2. Hummel KP, Dickie MM, Coleman DL: Diabetes, a new mutation in the mouse. *Science* 153:1127–1128, 1966.
3. Bray GA: The Zucker-fatty rat: A review. *Fed Proc* 36:148–153, 1977.
4. Michaelis OE, Patrick DH, Hansen CT, et al: Effect of dietary sucrose on the SHR-N-corpulent rat: A new model for insulin-independent diabetes. *Am J Clin Nutr* 39:612–618, 1984.
5. Russell JC, Amy RM: Early atherosclerotic lesions in a susceptible rat model: The LA/N-coruplent rat. *Atherosclerosis* 60:119–129, 1988.
6. Truett GE, Bahary N, Friedman JM, et al: Rat obesity gene fatty (fa) maps to chromosome 5: Evidence for homology with the mouse gene diabetes (db). *Proc Natl Acad Sci USA* 88:7806–7809, 1991.
7. Zucker LM, Antoniades HN: Insulin and obesity in the Zucker genetically obese rat "fatty." *Endocrinology* 90:1320–1330, 1972.
8. Phillips FC, Cleary MP: Metabolic measurements among homozygous (fa/fa) obese, heterozygous (Fa/fa) lean and homozygous (Fa/Fa) lean Zucker rat pups at 17 days of age. *J Nutr* 124:1230–1237, 1994.
9. Godbole V, York DA: Lipogenesis in situ in the genetically obese Zucker fatty rat (fa/fa): Role of hyperphagia and hyperinsulinaemia. *Diabetologia* 14:191–197, 1978.
10. Chan CP, Stern JS: Adipose lipoprotein lipase in insulin-treated diabetic lean and obese Zucker rats. *Am J Physiol* 242:E445–E450, 1982.
11. Penicaud L, Ferre P, Assimacopoulos-Jeannet F, et al: Increased gene expression of lipogenic enzymes and glucose transporter in white adipose tissue of suckling and weaned obese Zucker rats. *Biochem J* 279:303–308, 1991.
12. Kasiske BL, O'Donnell MP, Keane WF: The Zucker rat model of obesity,

insulin resistance, hyperlipidemia and renal injury. *Hypertension* 19: 1110–1115, 1992.

13. Briquet-Laugier V, Dugail I, Ardouin B, et al: Evidence for a sustained genetic effect on fat storage capacity in cultured adipose cells from Zucker rats. *Am J Physiol* 267:E439–E446, 1994.
14. Neely JR, Rovetto MJ, Oram FJ: Myocardial utilization of carbohydrate and lipids. *Prog Cardiovasc Dis* 15:289–329, 1972.
15. Reinauer H, Adrian M, Rösen P, et al: Influence of carnitine acyltransferase inhibitors on the performance and metabolism of rat cardiac muscle. *J Clin Chem Clin Biochem* 28:335–339, 1990.
16. Rösen P, Herberg L, Reinaur H: Different types of post-insulin receptor defects contribute to insulin resistance in hearts of obese Zucker rats. *Endocrinology* 119:1285–1291, 1986.
17. Lopaschuk GD, Belke DD, Gamble J, et al: Regulation of fatty acid oxidation in the mammalian heart in health and disease. *Biochim Biophys Acta* 1213:263–276, 1994.
18. Schulz H: Regulation of fatty acid oxidation in heart. *J Nutr* 124:165–171, 1994.
19. Quignard-Boulange A, Freyss-Beguin M, Brigant L, et al: Abnormal fatty acid utilization by cultured cardiac cells from 7-day-old obese Zucker rats. *J Cell Physiol* 140:449–454, 1989.
20. Randle PJ, Garland PB, Hales CN, et al: Interactions of metabolism and the physiological role of insulin. *Recent Prog Horm Res* 22:1–44, 1966.
21. Patten GS, Rattigan S, Filsell OH, et al: Insensitivity of cardiac phosphofructokinase to adrenergic activation in Zucker rats. *Biochem J* 218:483–488, 1984.
22. Ward WK, Beard JC, Halter JB, et al: Pathophysiology of insulin secretion in non-insulin-dependent diabetes mellitus. *Diabetes Care* 7:491–502, 1984.
23. Sanchez-Gutierrez JC, Sanchez-Arias JA, Lechuga CG, et al: Decreased responsiveness of basal gluconeogenesis to insulin action in hepatocytes isolated from genetically obese (fa/fa) Zucker rats. *Endocrinology* 134: 1868–1873, 1994.
24. Eckel J, Wirdeier A, Herberg L, et al: Insulin resistance in the heart: Studies on isolated cardiocytes of genetically obese Zucker rats. *Endocrinology* 116:1529–1534, 1985.
25. Zaninetti D, Greco-Perotto R, Assimacopoulos-Jeannet F, et al: Dysregulation of glucose transport and transporters in perfused hearts of genetically obese (fa/fa) rats. *Diabetologia* 32:56–60, 1989.
26. Uphues I, Kolter T, Goud B, et al: Failure of insulin regulated recruitment of the glucose transporter GLUT4 in cardiac muscle of obese Zucker rats is associated with alterations of small-molecular-mass GTP-binding proteins. *Biochem J* 311:161–166, 1995.
27. Slieker LJ, Roberts EF, Shaw WN, et al: Effect of streptozocin-induced diabetes on insulin-receptor tyrosine kinase activity in obese Zucker rats. *Diabetes* 39:619–625, 1990.
28. Van de Werve G, Zaninetti D, Michel U, et al: Identification of a major defect in insulin-resistant tissues of genetically obese (fa/fa) rats. *Diabetes* 36:310–314, 1987.
29. Alpert MA, Hashimi MW: Obesity and the heart. *Am J Med Sci* 306:117–123, 1993.

30. Paradise NF, Pilati CF, Payne WR, et al: Left ventricular function of the isolated, genetically obese rat's heart. *Am J Physiol* 248:H438–H444, 1985.
31. Segel LD, Rendig SV, Mason DT, et al: Isolated hearts from obese rats show impaired function during hypoxia. *Proc Soc Exp Biol Med* 163:111–119, 1980.
32. Paulson DJ, Tahiliano AG: Minireview: Cardiovascular abnormalities associated with human and rodent obesity. *Life Sci* 51:1557–1569, 1992.
33. Morris GS, Baldwin KM, Lash JM, et al: Exercise alters cardiac myosin isozyme distribution in obese Zucker and Wistar rats. *J Appl Physiol* 69:380–383, 1990.
34. Schaffer SW: Cardiomyopathy associated with noninsulin-dependent diabetes. *Mol Cell Biochem* 107:1–20, 1991.
35. Vernimmen C, Auclair MC, Lechat P: Reduced sensitivity of the heart ventricle of obese Zucker rats to isoprenaline. *C R Acad Sci III* 306:153–156, 1988.
36. Abel MA, Zemel MB: Impaired recovery of vascular smooth muscle intracellular calcium following agonist stimulation in insulin resistant (Zucker obese) rats. *Am J Hypertens* 6:500–504, 1993.
37. Hiramatsu S, Inoue K, Sako Y, et al: Secretion of insulin and glucagon by the perfused pancreas of genetically obese (fa/fa) Zucker rats and its alteration with aging. *Endocr J* 42:563–567, 1995.
38. Jeanrenaud B: Neuroendocrine and metabolic basis of type II diabetes as studied in animal models. *Diabetes Metab Rev* 4:603–614, 1988.
39. Chatelain P, Robberecht P, De Neef P, et al: Impairment of hormone-stimulated cardiac adenylate cyclase activity in the genetically obese (fa/fa) Zucker rat. *Pflugers Arch* 390:10–16, 1981.
40. Robberecht P, De Neef P, Camus JC, et al: The cardiac inotropic response to secretin is lower in genetically obese (fa/fa) than in lean (fa/?) Zucker rats. *Pflugers Arch* 398:217–220, 1983.
41. Strassheim D, Houslay MD, Milligan G: Regulation of cardiac adenylate cyclase activity in rodent models of obesity. *Biochem J* 283:203 208, 1992.
42. Bass S, Ritter S: Decreased β-adrenergic receptor binding in obese female Zucker rats. *J Autonom Nerv Syst* 14:81–87, 1985.
43. Auclair MC, Vernimmen C, Lavau M, et al: Dependence on extracellular potassium of the positive inotropic response to ST 587, a selective α-1 adrenoceptor agonist, in Zucker rat heart ventricle. *Life Sci* 44:1475–1482, 1989.

Chapter 3

Cardiac Morphology and Obesity in Man

Martin A. Alpert, MD
James K. Alexander, MD

Cardiac morphology in obese persons has been studied at necropsy by means of endomyocardial biopsy and with echocardiography. In this chapter we present a review and analysis of studies assessing cardiac morphology using these techniques in both adults and children with various degrees of obesity, and discuss the results of studies addressing the effects of weight loss on cardiac morphology in such individuals.

Postmortem and Endomyocardial Biopsy Studies

The first study to systemically characterize cardiac morphology in obese individuals was performed by Smith and Willius[1] and reported in 1933. Smith and Willius[1] analyzed postmortem findings in 135 patients who were 13% to 170% overweight. The study population included 4 morbidly obese individuals whose body weights ranged from 102 to 250 kg and who died of congestive heart failure (CHF). Most patients had underlying cardiovascular disease, including hypertension and coronary atherosclerosis. There was a linear increase in heart weight with increasing body weight up to 105 kg. Above this threshold, heart weight increased somewhat less in relation to body weight. The average heart weight was 444 g in men and 345 g in women. Both were substantially higher than the heart weight pre-

From: Alpert MA, and Alexander JK, (eds). *The Heart and Lung in Obesity*. Armonk, NY: Futura Publishing Company, Inc., © 1998.

dicted for individuals of comparable body height with normal body weight. The heart/body weight ratios were 0.41 in men and 0.35 in women, which were both lower than that of subjects with normal weight (0.43 for men and 0.40 for women). Smith and Willius[1] attributed the increase in heart weight to excessive epicardial fat, which was present in 95% of cases. Excessive epicardial fat was more prominent over the right ventricle. Isolated instances of penetration of epicardial fat into the right ventricular (RV) myocardium were identified. Such penetration of epicardial fat into the left ventricular (LV) myocardium was not observed. Intracellular fat content, based on microscopic analysis, was no greater in obese patients than in lean patients. This study is important primarily because it refuted the previously accepted hypothesis that obesity is commonly associated with fatty metamorphosis in myocardium and excessive intracellular accumulation of fat. Although, in retrospect, the authors overemphasized the importance of epicardial fat, their identification of 9 patients with CHF and no apparent underlying organic etiology (including 1 with massive biventricular hypertrophy) suggested the existence of a specific cardiomyopathy associated with obesity.

In 1968, Amad and colleagues[2] reported the results of a postmortem study of 12 predominately extremely obese patients (6 men and 6 women) who were normotensive and free from underlying organic heart disease during life. The amount over ideal body weight ranged from 34% to 240%. Three of 12 died of CHF. These investigators reported a direct linear correlation between body weight and heart weight, and between the increase in heart weight and body weight above predicted value. These findings confirmed the prior observations of Smith and Willius.[1] Heart weight was substantially higher than predicted for all 12 patients (410 to 1100 g). Nine of 12 patients had increased LV wall thickness and 2 had increased RV wall thickness. All patients studied had variable degrees of LV hypertrophy. One patient had interstitial fibrosis and 1 had focal perivascular fibrosis. Ten of 12 patients had normal amounts of epicardial fat. One patient had a slight increase and 1 had a moderate increase in epicardial fat. This is in contrast to the observations of Smith and Willius.[1] The coronary arteries were normal in 8 patients. Medial hypertrophy was noted in 2 patients, minimal intimal proliferation was observed in 1 patient and focal intimal fibrosis was present in 1 patient. The endocardium was normal in all patients studied. This study is important because it was the first to demonstrate that the increase in heart weight associated with obesity is due predominantly to ventricular (particularly LV) hypertrophy.

In 1967, Alexander and Pettigrove[3] reported the postmortem cardiac findings of nine patients whose body weight was 300 lbs or more. Eight of nine died with or from CHF. All nine had increased heart weight and all had LV hypertrophy, one patient had biventricular hypertrophy, and all patients were hypertensive. None of the patients had coronary artery disease (CAD) or valvular heart disease. Prior to this study, speculation existed that RV failure in extremely obese individuals occurred as an isolated phenomenon and resulted exclusively from pulmonary hypertension (cor pulmonale). This study demonstrated that CHF in such individuals usually evolves from LV hypertrophy and subsequent decompensation.

In 1984, Warnes and Roberts[4] reported cardiac findings in 12 (7 men and 5 women, 25 to 59 years old) massively obese patients studied at necropsy. Their body weight ranged from 312 to more than 500 lbs. Seven patients had systemic hypertension and 4 had sleep apnea/obesity hyperventilation syndrome. The causes of death were CHF in 2 patients, acute myocardial infarction in 1 patient, and aortic dissection in one patient. Five deaths were due to suicide, or were unexplained, and 3 were from noncardiac causes. The heart weight was increased in all patients (380 to 990 g). The heart/body weight ratio was 0.37, which was substantially lower than predicted. Unlike prior studies, there was no consistent relation between heart weight and body weight or between the increase in heart weight above predicted and the increase in body weight above ideal. The LV cavity was dilated in 11 patients, the RV cavity was dilated in all 12 patients, and the left atrial wall thickness was increased in all 12 patients. LV hypertrophy was symmetric in all patients and RV hypertrophy was present in 4 patients. Of 664 coronary artery segments studied, only 14% were narrowed more than 50% and only 3% were narrowed more than 75%. Evidence of myocardial necrosis or fibrosis was present in 2 patients. Subepicardial fat was increased in 9 patients (moderately in 4 and severely in 5) and RV fat infiltration was present in 3 patients. This study adds to our understanding of cardiac morphology in obesity by underscoring the ubiquitous presence of LV hypertrophy and the frequent presence of LV and RV dilatation in symptomatic morbidly obese individuals. This study also demonstrated that extremely obese patients who died prematurely did not have more coronary atherosclerosis than might be expected at their ages.

In 1992, Kasper et al.[5] reported the results of a study that compared myocardial biopsy findings in 43 obese patients with CHF and 409 lean patients with CHF. A specific cause of CHF (other than obesity) was identified in 64.5% of lean patients and in only 23.3% of obese patients, the majority of whom demonstrated myocardial hypertrophy.

These findings lend further credence to the concept of a specific cardiomyopathy associated with obesity.

Isolated case reports of postmortem findings in symptomatic morbidly obese patients have uniformly described the presence of LV dilatation and hypertrophy generally in association with RV dilatation and hypertrophy.[6–10]

Fatty Infiltration

Fatty infiltration of the heart is a condition in which epicardial fat extends into ventricular and atrial myocardium. It most frequently involves the right ventricle, perivascular region, and the cardiac skeleton. Until this century, fatty infiltration was considered a plausible explanation for sudden death based on the writings of such scholars as Celsus, Senac, Corvisart, and Laennec.[11–15] The overall incidence of fatty infiltration at autopsy has been estimated to be 3%.[11–16] Saphir and Corrigan[16] reviewed 58 cases in which fatty infiltration was found at necropsy. Eighteen patients were obese and 9 were emaciated. In all but 2 cases, fatty infiltration was considered to be an incidental finding, or at most a contributing factor to death. In 2 cases however (both obese women), death was sudden, unexpected, and not attributable to other identifiable causes. Subsequent case reports have described sinus node dysfunction or atrial fibrillation following fatty replacement of the sinus node in obese patients. Right bundle branch block, nonspecific intraventricular block, and complete heart block have been described in obese patients with fatty replacement/infiltration of the atrioventricular node or conduction fascicles.[17–19] Thus, fatty infiltration of the heart may rarely serve as a morphological substrate for sudden death in obese patients.

Smith and Willius[1] postulated that fatty infiltration of myocardium interfered with cardiac activity and nutrition, which was later proven erroneous. Carpenter[20] reviewed the clinical and postmortem findings of 52 patients with fatty infiltration and 52 controls of similar age and gender. Carpenter[20] identified two distinct patterns of fatty infiltration that he referred to as fatty metaplasia. The first pattern (uncomplicated fatty metaplasia) comprised cords of fat cells intermingled with small atrophic muscle bundles. Such cords frequently appeared to extend from epicardial fat. Similar findings were noted in control patients. The second pattern of fatty metaplasia comprised areas of fat surrounded by fibrosis and not attached to epicardial fat. The second form occurred most commonly in the setting of CAD. Obesity was not identified as a predictor of either form of fatty infiltration.

There is little evidence to implicate fatty infiltration as a cause of impaired cardiac function. A single case report by Dervan et al.[21] documents the presence of a restrictive cardiomyopathic hemodynamic pattern in a 57-year-old chronically obese man, in whom fatty infiltration of myocardium was documented by myocardial biopsy. However, this patient also had extensive coronary atherosclerosis and, in fact, required coronary artery bypass surgery. Thus, an ischemic etiology for both fatty infiltration and restrictive physiology cannot be excluded.

Echocardiographic Studies in Adults

Most information obtained from postmortem studies has been gleaned from patients who were severely obese during life. Many of these individuals suffered from CHF. Echocardiography has provided the opportunity to study various degrees of obesity and to assess cardiac morphology in asymptomatic individuals, as well as those with varying degrees of CHF. In doing so, these studies have confirmed, amplified, and extended the lessons learned from necropsy.

Incidence of Cardiac Chamber Enlargement and LV Hypertrophy

Relatively little information exists concerning the incidence of cardiac chamber enlargement and LV hypertrophy in obese individuals. In a study of 62 normotensive morbidly obese patients (mainly women) whose body weight was twice their ideal body weight or more, Alpert et al.[22] reported increased ventricular septal thickness in and/or LV posterior wall thickness in 56%, an increased LV internal dimension in diastole in 39%, increased LV mass in 64%, left atrial enlargement in 39%, and RV enlargement in 40%. Garcia et al.[23] studied 30 morbidly obese patients, of whom 15 were also hypertensive. LV end-diastolic volume was increased in 40%. LV mass was increased in 80%,[23] and left atrial enlargement was present in 40%. Both of these studies demonstrate that LV and RV enlargement, LV hypertrophy, and left atrial enlargement occur commonly in severely obese persons. Zema and Caccavano[24] studied 50 obese (predominately female) patients who were 59 to 60 inches tall and whose body weight ranged from 145 to 346 lbs. The study was originally designed to assess the feasibility of M-mode echocardiography in obese subjects and the authors made no attempt to exclude patients with underlying organic heart disease. LV dilatation was reported in 8% and LV hypertrophy was noted in 6%. The relatively low incidence of LV dilatation and hypertrophy compared with that noted in the previous studies of severely obese subjects may have resulted from a preponderance of mildly to moderately obese patients in the study population.

Comparison of LV Chamber Size, Wall Thickness, and Mass in Obese and Lean Persons

Five studies have compared LV chamber size, wall thickness, and LV mass in obese and lean subjects. The results of these studies are summarized in Table 1. The mean LV internal dimension in diastole, mean ventricular septal thickness, mean LV posterior wall thickness, and mean LV mass/height index, or mass index, were consistently significantly higher/greater in obese than in lean subjects in normotensive patients.[25–28] The mean LV radius to thickness ratio was significantly higher in obese than in lean subjects in one study[29] and not significantly different in obese and lean patients in another study.[27] In a study of normotensive mildly obese patients, the mean LV internal dimension in diastole, mean LV posterior wall thickness, mean ventricular septal thickness, and mean LV mass index were all significantly higher/greater in obese than in lean subjects.[29] These studies, together with the observations of Lauer et al.[30] indicate that obesity, regardless of severity, produces dilatation and hypertrophy of the LV. Since LV wall thickness is typically normal or only mildly increased, it is likely that dilatation precedes hypertrophy. Thus, LV hypertrophy associated with obesity is a form of eccentric hypertrophy.

Relation of Degree of Obesity To LV Mass and Dimension

Several studies have explored the relation of degree of obesity and LV mass. Lauer et al.[30] studied 3922 healthy participants of the Framingham Heart Study to assess the impact of mild to moderate obesity on LV mass and geometry. Body mass index correlated moderately and positively with LV mass in both men and women. After adjusting for age and blood pressure, body mass index remained a strong independent predictor of LV mass, LV wall thickness, and the LV internal dimension

Table 1
Echocardiographic Studies Assessing Left Ventricular Morphology in Normotensive Obese and Lean Patients

Key Variables	Studies				
	Merlino et al[25]	*Messerli et al[26]*	*Lavie et al[27]*	*Nakajima et al[28]*	*Ku et al[29]*
Number					
Obese	27	17	12	35	30
Lean	20	17	12	35	30
Gender					
Obese	12 women, 15 men	3 women, 14 men	Not provided	16 women, 19 men	15 women, 15 men
Lean	10 women, 10 men	3 women, 14 men		14 women, 16 men	15 women, 15 men
Mean age (years)					
Obese	36.2 ± 3.7	37 ± 8	34 ± 2	33.8 ± 8.6	20 ± 1
Lean	36.9 ± 3.5	34 ± 10	33 ± 3	34.5 ± 12.5	20 ± 1
Severity of obesity					
Obese	Moderate to severe BMI: 31.1 ± 5.6 kg/m²	Moderate 70 ± 22% OW	Moderate 71 ± 7% OW	Mild to moderate 47 ± 19% OW	Mild 76 ± 13 kg
Lean	BMI: 22.2 ± 2 kg/m²	−0.2 ± 6% OW	0.4 ± 1% OW	2 ± 6% OW	62 ± 8 kg
Mean LV internal dimension in diastole (cm)					
Obese	5.21 ± 0.50	5.95 ± 1.01	5.51 ± 0.27	5.5 ± 3.6	4.8 ± 0.8
Lean	4.95 ± 0.50	4.96 ± 0.62	4.91 ± 17	4.6 ± 2.3	4.4 ± 0.5
P	<0.02	<0.0001	<0.01	<0.001	<0.05
Mean ventricular septal thickness (cm)					
Obese	8.8 ± 1.8	1.21 ± 0.22	1.18 ± 0.07	9.1 ± 0.6	1.0 ± 0.7

Table 1—Continued

Key Variables	Studies				
	Merlino et al[25]	Messerli et al[26]	Lavie et al[27]	Nakajima et al[28]	Ku et al[29]
Lean	8.0 ± 1.3	0.93 ± 0.20	0.92 ± 0.05	8.5 ± 0.4	8.3 ± 0.3
P	N.S.	<0.0001	<0.01	<0.001	<0.01
Mean LV posterior wall thickness (cm)					
Obese	—	1.16 ± 0.23	1.11 ± 0.07	9.5 ± 0.9	10.8 ± 0.2
Lean	—	0.89 ± 0.16	0.90 ± 0.14	8.8 ± 0.7	8.8 ± 0.4
P	—	<0.0001	<0.01	<0.001	<0.001
Mean LV mass (g)					
Obese	182.3 ± 96.3	367.6 ± 177.4	317.9 ± 34.2	—	181 ± 6
Lean	134.9 ± 35.5	199.9 ± 67.4	200.2 ± 21.6	—	122 ± 7
P	<0.003	<0.001	<0.01	—	<0.001
Mean LV mass index (g/m²)					
Obese	—	119.4 ± 44.4	147.8 ± 15.5	—	98 ± 3
Lean	—	79.5 ± 82.7	115.0 ± 13.9	—	71 ± 4
P	—	<0.002	—	—	<0.001
Mean LV mass/height index (g/m)					
Obese	112.1 ± 32.9	—	—	—	—
Lean	84.3 ± 25.1	—	—	—	—
P	<0.02	—	—	—	—
LV radius/thickness ratio					
Obese	—	2.62 ± 0.52	—	2.80 ± 0.13	—
Lean	—	2.85 ± 0.61	—	2.69 ± 0.13	—
P	—	N.S.	—	<0.01	—

LV = left ventricular; BMI = body mass index; OW = overweight.

in diastole. The prevalence of LV hypertrophy was particularly high in subjects whose body mass index was greater than 30 kg/m^2 (32% in men and 30% in women). Similarly, de la Maza and coworkers[31] noted a significantly positive correlation between LV mass and body mass index in 29 normotensive and 21 hypertensive moderately obese subjects. In a study of 25 obese men whose body weight ranged from 62.2 to 128.6 kg and whose body mass index ranged from 20.9 to 44.5 kg/m^2. Rasooly and colleagues[32] reported strong positive correlations between LV mass and both waist circumference and waist/hip ratio. A recent study of 50 morbidly obese (twice their ideal body weight or more) subjects (80% women) by Alpert and coworkers[33] demonstrated a significant positive correlation between percent overweight and LV mass/height index (Figure 1). These studies confirm that increasing severity of central obesity is associated with progressive augmentation of LV mass, thus extending the work of Smith and Willius.[1]

Other Factors Contributing to LV Hypertrophy in Obese Persons

Several studies have identified additional factors that may contribute to the development of eccentric LV hypertrophy in obese patients. These include: unfavorable alterations in LV loading conditions (including hypertension), duration of obesity, and possibly insulin resistance.

In a study of 50 normotensive asymptomatic morbidly obese subjects (80% women), Alpert et al.[27] reported significant positive correlations between LV mass/height index and the LV internal dimension in diastole (an index of preload), systolic blood pressure, and LV end-systolic wall stress (indices of afterload) (Figure 1). This study suggests that unfavorable alterations in LV loading conditions contribute directly to the development of LV hypertrophy in severely obese subjects. Unfortunately, similar studies have not been performed on mildly and moderately obese subjects. Hypertension in particular is a major determinant of LV hypertrophy in obese individuals. In a comparison of normotensive and hypertensive moderately obese and lean subjects, Messerli and coworkers[26] found that the mean LV internal dimension in diastole, mean LV mass, mean LV mass index, and mean left atrial dimension were all greater in hypertensive obese and lean patients than in their corresponding normotensive counterparts. As was noted in normotensive patients, mean values for these variables in hypertensive patients were significantly greater in obese than in lean subjects.

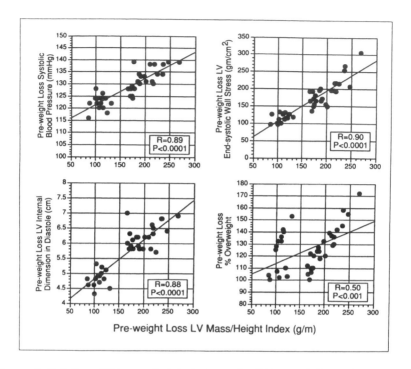

Pre-weight Loss LV Mass/Height Index (g/m)

Figure 1. Relation of LV mass/height index to the LV internal dimension in diastole, systolic blood pressure, and LV end-systolic wall stress in morbidly obese patients. LV mass/height index correlated positively and significantly with each of these variables. (Reproduced from *Am J Cardiol* 73:918–921, 1994 with permission.)

In a report assessing separate and joint influences of obesity and mild hypertension on LV mass and geometry derived from the Framingham Heart Study, Lauer and coworkers[34] showed that obesity and hypertension each have distinct associations with LV mass and diastolic dimension that are additive, but not synergistic.

Two studies have assessed the relation of duration of obesity and LV morphology.[28,35] A study of 50 morbidly obese patients (40 women and 10 men), by Alpert et al.,[35] reported significant positive correlations between duration of morbid obesity and LV mass/height index (Figure 2). Duration of morbid obesity also correlated significantly and positively with the LV internal dimension in diastole, systolic blood pressure, and LV end-systolic wall stress (Figure 2).[34] Nakajima and colleagues[28] had previously reported that the mean LV internal dimension index in diastole and radius/thickness ratio were significantly greater in 17 mildly to moderately obese patients who were obese for longer

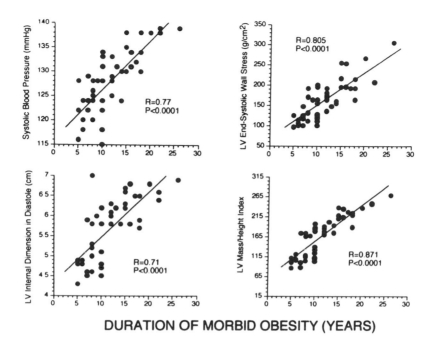

DURATION OF MORBID OBESITY (YEARS)

Figure 2. Relation of duration of morbid obesity to LV mass/height index, the LV internal dimension in diastole, systolic blood pressure, and LV end-systolic wall stress. Duration of morbid obesity correlated positively and significantly with each of these variables. (Reproduced from *Am J Cardiol* 76.1194–1197, 1995 with permission.)

than 15 years than in 18 patients who had been mildly to moderately obese for 15 years or less. Thus, duration of obesity appears to be an important determinant of LV chamber size and mass in obese persons. However, it is not clear whether this influence is independent of LV loading conditions.

Sasson and coworkers[36] explored the intriguing possibility of a relation between insulin resistance and echocardiographic LV hypertrophy in 40 normotensive, nondiabetic healthy obese adults. Insulin resistance was assessed by obtaining plasma glucose and insulin levels during an intravenous glucose tolerance test, which evaluated insulin integration over 90 minutes and determined the rate of glucose disposal. Multivariate regression analysis showed that LV mass correlated positively and significantly with plasma insulin levels at 90 minutes and the rate of glucose disposal independent of body mass index or blood pressure. The results suggest that insulin resistance may be an important determinant of LV mass in obese, normotensive nondiabetics. The authors of this study postulated that enhanced activity of insulin-like growth factor 1 may account for these observations.

Comparative Cardiac Morphology in Patients With and Without CHF

Most of the necropsy studies previously discussed included severely obese patients with CHF during life. All demonstrated LV enlargement and hypertrophy (often massive), as well as frequent left atrial and RV enlargement in such individuals. However, necropsy studies comparing obese patients with and without CHF are lacking. To assess the comparative cardiac morphology in obese patients with and without CHF, Alpert et al.[37] studied 74 normotensive morbidly obese subjects: 24 with and 50 without CHF. Approximately 80% of those studied in both groups were women. All were free from organic heart disease unrelated to obesity. Both the mean LV internal dimension in diastole and mean LV mass/height index were significantly greater in patients with than in those without CHF. In addition, mean left atrial and mean RV dimensions were significantly greater in patients with than in those without CHF. Mean duration of severe obesity, mean systolic blood pressure, and mean LV end-systolic wall stress were significantly higher/greater in those with than in those without CHF. This suggests that the comparatively greater LV mass/height index in those with CHF is due to longer duration of morbid obesity, more severely adverse alterations in LV loading conditions, or both.

Echocardiographic Studies in Children

Several studies have addressed the issue of cardiac morphology in obese children.[38–42] DeSimone et al.[38] reported a significant positive correlation between LV mass and body weight in 61 children and adults. The correlation was weaker, but still significant using body mass index. In a study of 341 children, including 106 6-year-olds, 166 12-year-olds, and 64 15-year-olds by Kono and coworkers,[39] the obesity index correlated strongly and positively with both the LV internal dimension in diastole and LV mass as early as age 6. In contrast, Yoshinaga and colleagues[40] found no correlation between LV wall thickness and indices of obesity in their study of 267 12-year-old boys and girls. Similarly, Koehler and coworkers[41] reported no correlation between the amount overweight and LV mass in 46 moderately obese children. These studies indicate that a variable relation exists between indices of body weight/obesity and both LV chamber size and LV mass.

In a study by Daniels et al.,[42] lean body mass resulting from linear growth was found to be the predominant factor in determining LV mass with fat mass and systolic blood pressure of lesser importance. Thus, in normal children and adolescents the impact of fat mass may be small with its major effects possibly mediated through alterations in lean body mass.

Controlled studies provide compelling evidence of an adverse effect of obesity on LV morphology. In one study, normalized LV mass was significantly higher in six obese boys and eight obese girls than in 139 lean boys and 114 lean girls, respectively.[39] In another study of 45 obese children (49% to 144% overweight) and 20 normal controls, the mean LV dimension in diastole, mean septal thickness, mean posterior LV wall thickness, and mean LV mass were all significantly greater in obese than in lean children.[40] The results of these studies suggest that obesity in children produces dilatation of the LV and a subsequent increase in LV mass in a manner similar to that described in adults.

Effect of Weight Loss on Cardiac Morphology

An increasing body of evidence suggests that weight reduction may produce favorable alterations in LV morphology. Six studies involving mildly, moderately, and severely obese subjects address this issue. The results of these studies are shown in Table 2.

Alpert and coworkers[22] used echocardiography to define LV morphology before and after weight loss in 34 morbidly obese patients. They demonstrated that substantial weight loss induced by vertical band gastroplasty produced a significant reduction in the mean LV internal dimension in diastole in those with LV enlargement prior to weight loss, but not in those with normal LV cavity size prior to weight loss. Weight loss produced no significant changes in mean ventricular septal thickness, mean posterior LV wall thickness, mean left atrial dimension, or mean RV internal dimension in either group. In a follow-up study, Alpert and coworkers[43] found that substantial weight loss produced significant reductions of both the mean LV internal dimension in diastole and mean LV mass/height index in those with increased LV mass/height index prior to weight loss, but no significant change in those whose pre-weight loss LV mass/height index was normal. The

Table 2
Effect of Weight Loss On Left Ventricular Morphology: Echocardiographic Studies

Variable	Alpert et al[22]		Alpert et al[43]		McMahon et al[44]	Wirth et al[45]		Himeno et al[46]		Jordan et al[47]
	Normal	Enlarged	Normal	Increased		Diet Alone	Diet and Exercise	Normotensive	Hypertensive	
Number of patients	34		14	25	15	22	21	11	11	14
Gender distribution male/female	2/32		12/2	21/4	4/11	12/31		2/9	2/9	—
Mean age (years)	38 ± 4		37 ± 8		39.3 ± 10.6	46 ± 8	44 ± 7	35 ± 7	37 ± 11	—
Weight loss modality	Gastroplasty		Gastroplasty		Diet	Diet and Diet	Exercise	Diet and Exercise		Sertaline and Diet
Severity of obesity	Severe		Severe		Moderate	Moderate		Mild to Moderate		Mild to Moderate
Before	135 ± 8 kg		130% ± 7% overweight		BMI: 31.8 ± 3.8 kg/m²	Weight: 95 ± 10 kg	Weight: 96 ± 11 kg	BMI: 30.7 ± 2.7 kg/m²	BMI: 31.9 ± 4.3 kg/m²	BMI: 36 ± 6 kg/m²
After	79 ± 6 kg		38% ± 6% overweight		BMI: 29.0 ± 4.2 kg/m²	Weight 88 ± 9 kg <0.001	Weight: 90 ± 11 kg <0.01	BMI: 28.8 ± 2.7 kg/m²	BMI: 30.2 ± 4.0 kg/m²	BMI: 34 ± 6 kg/m²
LVIDd (cm)										
Before	5.1 ± 0.3	6.0 ± 0.3	5.1 ± 0.4	6.2 ± 0.4	51.3 ± 6.1	5.35 ± 0.47	5.29 ± 0.33	4.70 ± 0.35	4.90 ± 0.36	5.3 ± 6.0
After	5.1 ± 0.2	5.1 ± 0.3	5.0 ± 0.3	5.7 ± 0.3	50.5 ± 6.1	5.37 ± 5.06	5.06 ± 0.35	4.70 ± 0.40	5.08 ± 0.42	5.2 ± 6.0
p	N.S.	<0.02	N.S.	<0.001	—	<0.05	<0.001	N.S.	N.S.	N.S.

Ventricular septal thickness (cm)										
Before	0.9 ± 0.1	1.3 ± 0.1	—	—	8.9 ± 1.7	8.8 ± 1.4	9.8 ± 1.1	0.93 ± 0.19	0.89 ± 0.12	11.1 ± 2.0
After	0.9 ± 0.1	1.3 ± 0.1	—	—	7.7 ± 1.5	8.5 ± 1.4	8.8 ± 1.2	0.84 ± 0.15	0.8N± 0.12	10.5 ± 1.0
p	N.S.	N.S.	—	—	<0.05	<0.05	N.S.	<0.02	N.S.	N.S.
LV posterior Wall thickness (cm)										
Before	0.9 ± 0.1	1.3 ± 0.1	—	—	8.5 ± 1.7	9.3 ± 1.2	9.8 ± 1.1	1.02 ± 0.12	1.06 ± 0.15	11.1 ± 2.0
After	0.9 ± 0.1	1.3 ± 0.1	—	—	7.6 ± 1.8	9.2 ± 1.3	9.5 ± 1.2	0.98 ± 0.14	0.88 ± 0.14	10.0 ± 1.0
p	N.S.	N.S.	—	—	—	N.S.	<0.05	N.S.	N.S.	N.S.
LV mass (g)										
Before	—	—	—	—	193.0 ± 60.7	238 ± 57	244 ± 46	—	—	232 ± 62
After	—	—	—	—	155.2 ± 46.0	227 ± 48	219 ± 38	—	—	202 ± 43
p	—	—	—	—	—	<0.05	<0.001	—	—	<0.008
LVMHI (g/m)										
Before	—	—	138 ± 35	219 ± 22	—	—	—	—	—	—
After	—	—	105 ± 21	150 ± 17	—	—	—	—	—	—
p	—	—	N.S.	<0.0001	—	—	—	—	—	—
LVMI (g/m²)										
Before	—	—	—	—	92.4 ± 25.5	—	—	—	—	107 ± 27
After	—	—	—	—	77.6 ± 21.7	—	—	—	—	95 ± 17
p	—	—	—	—	—	—	—	—	—	<0.04

LV = left ventricular; LVIDd = left ventricular internal dimension in diastole; LVIMHI = left ventricular mass/height index; BMI = body mass index. Data are expressed as mean values ± 1 standard deviation.

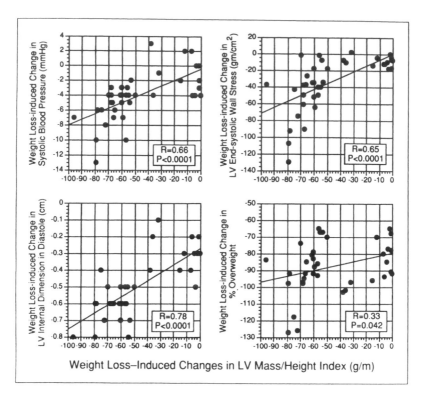

Weight Loss–Induced Changes in LV Mass/Height Index (g/m)

Figure 3. Relation of weight loss-induced change in LV mass/height index to the change in percent overweight and weight loss-induced changes in the LV internal dimension in diastole, systolic blood pressure, and LV end-systolic wall stress in morbidly obese patients. The magnitude of change (decrease) in LV mass/height correlated positively and significantly with the weight loss-induced changes (decreases) in each of these variables. (Reproduced from *Am J Cardiol* 73:918–921, 1994 with permission.)

magnitude of weight loss-induced change (decrease) in ventricular mass/height index correlated positively and significantly with the magnitude with weight loss-induced changes (decreases) in the percent overweight, the LV internal dimension in diastole, systolic blood pressure, and LV end-systolic wall stress (Figure 3).[43] Weight loss-induced alterations in LV morphology were assessed an average of 4.1 months after surgery.[43] The results of these studies show that in morbidly obese individuals substantial weight loss is capable of producing significant reductions in LV chamber size and mass in severely obese individuals. Such alterations occur primarily in those with eccentric LV hypertrophy prior to weight loss. Reduction of LV chamber size and mass in the morbidly obese occurs relatively soon after weight loss and appears to be related in part to favorable alterations in LV loading conditions.

Weight loss also appears to alter LV morphology favorably in mildly to moderately obese persons. MacMahon et al.[44] studied 41 mildly to moderately overweight, hypertensive patients using echocardiography to determine the effect of weight reduction on LV mass. Fifteen patients were studied before and after dietary weight reduction and were compared with 14 patients treated with metoprolol and 12 patients treated with a placebo.[44] After 28 weeks, those in the weight reduction group had lost 8.3 kg. This was accompanied by significant decreases in mean ventricular septal thickness, mean LV posterior wall thickness, LV mass, and LV mass index. The observed changes were accompanied by a significant decrease in diastolic, but not systolic blood pressure. In contrast, metoprolol produced no significant changes in mean LV cavity size, wall thickness, or mass despite (nonsignificant) reductions in systolic and diastolic pressure. Placebo produced no significant changes in any variable studied. This study was the first to show that weight loss in mildly and moderately obese patients is capable of reducing LV mass independent of blood pressure and heart rate. Similar findings were noted by Wirth and Kröger[45] in an echocardiographic study of 43 moderately obese patients whose weight loss was achieved using a hypocaloric diet (800 kcal/d) with or without regular aerobic exercise, by Himeno and colleagues[46] in a study of 22 moderately obese normotensive and hypertensive patients treated with a hypocaloric diet plus exercise, and by Jordan and coworkers[47] who used sertraline to facilitate dietary weight loss.

These studies demonstrate that weight reduction in mildly to moderately obese persons is capable of reducing LV cavity size and LV mass. In contrast to the studies of Alpert et al. in morbidly obese patients, morphological alterations in mildly to moderately obese persons occurred independent of blood pressure. The variable effect of weight loss on LV cavity size and wall thickness may relate to the relative influence of afterload and preload reduction.

Summary

In summary, LV enlargement and eccentric LV hypertrophy are the most common cardiac morphological abnormalities in obese individuals. Left atrial enlargement occurs frequently. The presence and degree of

LV dilatation and hypertrophy depend on severity and duration of obesity, and on the influence of adverse loading conditions. LV dilatation and hypertrophy are nearly ubiquitous in morbidly obese patients who have died with or from CHF. LV dilatation and hypertrophy are somewhat less common in asymptomatic morbidly obese patients. In mildly to moderately obese persons, LV mass and chamber size are greater than in matched controls. Studies of obese children indicate that these morphological changes may occur as early as 6 years of age. RV dilatation is much more common in symptomatic severely obese patients, but is less frequently encountered in asymptomatic obese persons. RV hypertrophy is less common than LV hypertrophy in obese patients. Weight loss consistently produces a decrease in LV mass, regardless of severity of obesity, particularly, and perhaps exclusively, in those with LV hypertrophy prior to weight loss. The effect of weight loss on LV cavity size and wall thickness is more variable. Whether weight loss-related reduction of LV chamber size and regression of LV hypertrophy may occur independent of loading conditions is uncertain. Weight loss related alterations in preload and afterload appear to be important determinants of the effect of weight loss on LV morphology. In less severely obese patients afterload may be a less important determinant of LV morphology after weight loss. Little information exists concerning the effect of weight loss on left atrial and right heart morphology. Fatty infiltration is more common in morbidly obese than in mildly obese, moderately obese, and lean individuals, but is not unique to obese individuals.

References

1. Smith HL, Willius FA: Adiposity of the heart. *Arch Intern Med* 52:929–931, 1933.
2. Amad KH, Brennan JC, Alexander JK: The cardiac pathology of obesity. *Circulation* 32:740–745, 1968.
3. Alexander JK, Pettigrove JK: Obesity and congestive heart failure. *Geriatrics* 22:101–108, 1967.
4. Warnes CA, Roberts WC: The heart in massive (more than 300 pounds or 136 kilograms) obesity. Analysis of 12 patients studied at necropsy. *Am J Cardiol* 54:1087–1091, 1984.
5. Kasper EK, Hruban RH, Baughman KL: Cardiomyopathy of obesity: A clinico-pathologic evaluation of 43 obese patients with heart failure. *Am J Cardiol* 70:921–924, 1992.
6. Counihan TB: Heart failure due to extreme obesity. *Br Heart J* 18:425–426, 1956.
7. Seide MJ: Heart failure due to extreme obesity. Report of a case with autopsy findings. *N Engl J Med* 251:1227–1230, 1957.

8. Clinicopathologic Conference—Barnes Hospital: Massive obesity and cardiac failure.*Am J Med* 64:827–833, 1978.
9. Carroll D: A peculiar type of cardiopulmonary failure associated with obesity. *Am J Med* 21:819–824, 1956.
10. Lillington GA, Anderson MA, Brandenberg RO: The cardiorespiratory syndrome of obesity. *Dis Chest* 32:1–20, 1957.
11. Bedford E: The story of fatty heart. A disease of Victorian times. *Br Heart J* 34:23–28, 1972.
12. Sprengell CJ: The aphorisms of Hippocrates and the sentences of Celsus. Boawick, London, 1708.
13. Senac JB: *Traifé de la structure du coeur, de son action, et de ses,* Maladies 2nd edition, Volume 2. Mequigron, Paris, 1783, p. 384.
14. Corvisart JN: *Ensai sur les maladies et les lesions organiques du coeur et des gros vaisseaus.* Migreret, Paris, 1806.
15. Laennec RTH: *De l'auscultation médiaté ou traité due diagnostique des madadies des poupons et du coeur* (volume 2). Brossin and Chaudé, Paris, 1819, p. 295.
16. Saphir O, Corrigan M: Fatty infiltration of myocardium. *Arch Intern Med* 52:410–428, 1933.
17. Case records, Massachusetts General Hospital 251:660–664, 1954.
18. Balsaver AM, Morales AR, Whitehouse FW: Fat infiltration of myocardium as a course of a cardiac conduction defect. *Am J Cardiol* 19:261–266, 1967.
19. Spain DM, Cathcart RT: Heart block caused by fat infiltration of the interventricular septum "cor adiposum". *Am Heart J* 32:659–664, 1946.
20. Carpenter HM: Myocardial fat infiltration. *Am Heart J* 63:491–496, 1962.
21. Dervain JP, Ilercit A, Kane PB, et al: Fatty infiltration: Another restrictive cardiomyopathy pattern. *Cathet Cardiovasc Diagn* 22:184–189, 1991.
22. Alpert MA, Terry BE, Kelly DK: Effect of weight loss on cardiac chamber size, wall thickness and left ventricular function in morbid obesity. *Am J Cardiol* 55:783–786, 1985.
23. Garcia LC, Laredo C, Arriaga J, et al: Echocardiographic findings in obesity. *Rev Invest Clin* 34:235–242, 1982.
24. Zema MJ, Caccavano M: Feasibility of detailed M-mode echocardiographic examination in markedly obese adults: Prospective study of 50 patients. *J Clin Ultrasound* 10:31–34, 1982.
25. Merlino G, Scaglione R, Corrao S, et al: Association between reduced lymphocyte beta-adrenergic receptors and left ventricular dysfunction in young obese subjects. *Int J Obes* 18:699–703, 1994.
26. Messerli FII, Sungaard-Rilse ED, Dreslinski GR, et al: Dimorphic cardiac adaptation to obesity and arterial hypertension. *Ann Intern Med* 94:757–761, 1983.
27. Lavie CJ, Amodeo C, Ventura HO, et al: Left atrial abnormalities indicating diastolic ventricular dysfunction in cardiomyopathy of obesity. *Chest* 92:1042–1046, 1987.
28. Nakajima T, Fuhoka S, Tokunaga K, et al: Noninvasive study of left ventricular performance in obese patients: Influences of duration of obesity. *Circulation* 71:481–486, 1985.
29. Ku C, Lin S, Wang D, et al: Left ventricular filling in normotensive obese adults. *Am J Cardiol* 73:613–615, 1994.
30. Lauer MS, Anderson KM, Kannel WB: The impact of obesity on left ven-

tricular mass and geometry. The Framingham Study. *JAMA* 266:231–236, 1991.

31. de la Maza MP, Estevez A, Bunoat D, et al: Ventricular mass in hypersensitive and normotensive obese subjects. *Int J Obes* 18:193–197, 1994.
32. Rasooly Y, Sasson Z, Gupta R: Relation between body fat distribution and left ventricular mass in men without structural heart disease or systemic hypertension. *Am J Cardiol* 71:1477–1479, 1993.
33. Alpert MA, Lambert CR, Terry BE, et al: Interrelationship of left ventricular mass systolic function and diastolic filling in normotensive morbidly obese patients. *Int J Obes* 19:550–557, 1995.
34. Lauer MS, Anderson KM, Levy D: Separate and joint influences of obesity and mild hypertension on left ventricular mass and geometry: The Framingham Heart Study. *JACC* 19:130–134, 1992.
35. Alpert MA, Lambert CR, Panayiotou H, et al: Relationship of duration of morbid obesity to left ventricular mass, systolic function and diastolic filling and effect of weight loss. *Am J Cardiol* 76:1194–1197, 1995.
36. Sasson Z, Rasooly Y, Bhesania T, et al: Insulin resistance is an important determinant of left ventricular mass in obese. *Circulation* 88:1431–1436, 1993.
37. Alpert MA, Terry BE, Mulekar M, et al: Cardiac morphology and left ventricular function in morbidly obese patients with and without congestive heart failure and effect of weight loss. *Am J Cardiol,* in press.
38. DeSimone G, Daniels SR, Devereux RB, et al: Left ventricular mass and body size in normotensive children and adults: Assessment of allometric relations and impact of overweight. *J Am Coll Cardiol* 20:1251–1260, 1992.
39. Kono Y, Yoshinaga M, Oku S, et al: Effect of obesity on echocardiographic parameters in children. *Int J Cardiol* 46:773, 1994.
40. Yoshinaga M, Yuasa Y, Hatano H, et al: Effect of total adipose weight and systemic hypertension on left ventricular mass in children. *Am J Cardiol* 76:785–787, 1995.
41. Kochler B, Maleck-Tendera E, Drzewiecka B, et al: Evaluation of the cardiovascular system in children with simple obesity: Part II. Echocardiographic assessment. *Materia Med Polona* 2:131–133, 1989.
42. Daniels SR, Kimball TR, Morrison JA, et al: Effect of lean body mass, fat mass, blood pressure and sexual maturation on left ventricular mass in children and adolescents. *Circulation* 92:3249–3254, 1995.
43. Alpert MA, Lambert CR, Terry BE, et al: Effect of weight loss on left ventricular mass in nonhypertensive morbidly obese patients. *Am J Cardiol* 73:918–921, 1994.
44. MacMahon SW, Wilcken DEL, MacDonald GJ: The effect of weight reduction on left ventricular mass. A randomized, controlled trial in young, overweight, hypertensive patients. *N Engl J Med* 314:334–339, 1986.
45. Wirth A, Kröger H: Improvement of left ventricular morphology and function in obese subjects following a diet and exercise program. *Int J Obes* 19:61–66, 1995.
46. Himeno E, Nishino K, Nakashima Y, et al: Weight reduction regresses left ventricular mass regardless of blood pressure level in obese subjects. *Am Heart J* 131:313–319, 1996.
47. Jordan J, Messerli FH, Lavie CJ, et al: Reduction of weight and left ventricular mass with serotonin uptake inhibition in obese patients with systemic hypertension. *Am J Cardiol* 75:743–747, 1995.

Chapter 4

Hemodynamic Alterations with Obesity in Man

James K. Alexander, MD
Martin A. Alpert, MD

This chapter reviews and analyzes studies assessing central and peripheral hemodynamics with obesity at rest, during exercise, and following weight loss, and considers both normotensive and hypertensive subjects. Insofar as possible, the degree of obesity is related to the extent to hemodynamic alteration.

Hemodynamics in Normotensive Obese Subjects

Increases in body oxygen consumption, blood volume, and cardiac output, as measured by the direct Fick method, parallel the amount of overweight in normotensive morbidly obese subjects at rest (Figure 1).[1–5] Comparable increments in cardiac output have also been found to utilize the thermodilution method.[6,7] As heart rate remains at normal levels, stroke volume and left ventricular (LV) stroke work are also elevated. These same positive correlations among blood volume, cardiac output, and stroke volume with body mass index (BMI), or relative body weight (RBW), also obtain in mildly overweight (RBW 114.3% ± 1.5%, moderately obese (RBW 148.7% ± 12.1%),[9] and markedly obese (RBW 172.2% ± 6.5%)[10] subjects using indocyanine green dye for estimation of cardiac output or radionuclide angiocardiography in the latter group (BMI 35.1 ± 5.6).[11] Echocardiographic studies of moderately obese (RBW 147% ± 19%)[12] or mildly to markedly obese (RBW 120% to 190%)[13] subjects have

From: Alpert MA, and Alexander JK, (eds). *The Heart and Lung in Obesity.* Armonk, NY: Futura Publishing Company, Inc., © 1998.

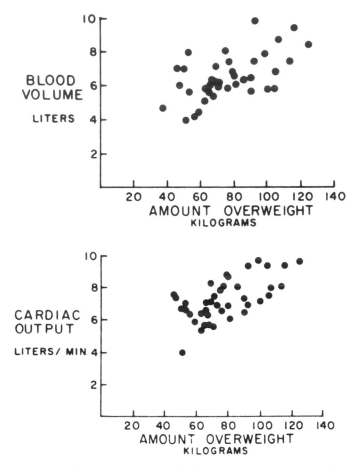

Figure 1. Relation of the amount overweight to oxygen consumption, blood volume, and cardiac output. Increases in the amount overweight are paralleled by increases in blood volume and cardiac output. (Reproduced from Reference 1 with permission.)

reaffirmed the correlations among LV preload, stroke volume, and cardiac output with increasing weight gain. When patients are 100 kg overweight, resting cardiac output may be as much as 10 L/min, or twice that at ideal weight.[2] Thus, morbid obesity leads to a high cardiac output state, with lowered systemic vascular resistance in normotensive subjects.

Since systemic arteriovenous oxygen content difference is usually slightly widened, reflecting a lesser oxygen extraction by adipose tissue than other parenchymal organs, blood flow per unit body weight is reduced (vide infra).[14] In contrast to these hemodynamic findings with increase in total fat mass, central obesity or excess abdominal fat, as defined by waist/hip ratio, is characterized by higher total peripheral vascular resistance and lower cardiac output.[15] However, in both markedly obese subjects with predominantly peripheral obesity (BMI 33.5 ± 4 kg/m^2, waist/hip ratio 0.87 ± 0.04) or combined peripheral and central obesity (BMI 35.9 ± 5.9 kg/m^2, waist/hip ratio 0.97 ± 0.07), cardiac output, stroke volume, and LV volumes are increased.[16]

Peripheral Hemodynamics with Obesity

Limited information is available relative to the regional distribution of blood flow in the high cardiac state characterizing marked obesity. Estimation of cerbral blood flow (CBF) by the nitrous oxide method in 14 extremely obese normotensive adults (RBW 183% to 279%) yielded a mean of 59 ± 10 mL per 100 g/min at rest,[17] approximating a "normal" level of 54 ± 12 mL per 100 g/min reported by Kety and Schmidt[18] and others.[17] Since a survey of brain weight at autopsy in 21 obese subjects yielded a mean value of 1341, with a range of 1100 to 1570 g,[17] the usually assumed normal adult brain weight of 1400 g was taken for extrapolation of total cerebral flow to 809 ± 167 mL/min, again not significantly different from the mean value of 750 mL/min found in normal adults.[18] CBF accounted by 13% of cardiac output (Fick method), somewhat lower than the normal value of 16%.[18] Cerebral oxygen uptake (3.1 ± 0.7 mL per 100 g/min) and total cerebral oxygen consumption (43 ± 8 mL O$_2$/min) were within a normal range.[18] However, cerebral percentages of cardiac output and body oxygen uptake were reduced from normal values of 16% and 24% to 13% and 16%, respectively. Splanchnic blood flow estimates in 11 of these subjects, using the sulfobromophthalein extraction method,[19] were higher than predicted normal at ideal weight (1451 mL/min vs. 1145).[17] However, the increases in splanchnic flow over predicted normal, ranging from 30 to 800 mL/min, were not sufficient to account for increments in cardiac output over predicted normal at ideal weight, which has sometimes been as great as 4 to 5 L/min. Renal plasma and blood flow measurements in 12 of these subjects from the clearance of para-aminohippuric acid were low normal as compared with those at predicted ideal weight (449 ± mL/min vs. 549, and 741 ± 195 mL/min vs. 911, respectively). Renal blood flow as a percentage of cardiac output, 11.4% ± 2.3%, as compared with the predicted normal of 18%, was significantly reduced. A subsequent study demonstrated no significant difference in renal blood flow between lean and obese (RBW 172%) subjects.[20] Although blood flow to resting muscle and skin has not been quantitated in obese subjects, and increased muscle mass may be present, it does not appear that resting muscle blood flow could account for the increases in cardiac output reaching levels of 10 L/min.[1] Adipose tissue blood flow, as estimated by inert gas studies averages 2 to 3 mL/min per 100 g under resting conditions.[21] Thus, 100 kg of fat would require as much as 3 L/min blood flow. Since the large increments in cardiac output with extreme obesity cannot be accounted for by flow to other parenchymal organs, it may be concluded that the high output state of obesity results largely from the requirement of adipose tissue blood flow. However, since blood flow per unit tissue weight of adipose tissue is less than that of other organs, cardiac output per kilogram body weight is less in obese subjects than those at ideal weight.[1] These changes in blood volume and flow are accompanied by increments in intracardiac pressures in normotensive morbidly obese subjects. At rest, LV and right ventricular (RV) end-diastolic, pulmonary wedge, and pulmonary artery pressures tend to be at upper normal level or elevated.[2–7,14] With exercise, augmentation of cardiac output is appropriate for lower workloads, but falls off at higher loads. That is, with increases in body oxygen uptake two to three times the resting level, the relation between cardiac output increment and oxygen uptake (the so-called exercise factor) is well within the normal range,[2,4] but when oxygen uptake increases to five times the resting level, it falls to a low normal level.[3] Increase in cardiac output with exercise is accomplished at the expense of augmented LV filling pressure. In virtually all cases LV end-diastolic pressures rise to abnormal levels and frequently as high as 20 to 35 mm Hg,[4,12] with accompanying increments in pulmonary wedge, pulmonary artery, and RV end-diastolic pressures.[2–4,7] Although moderate increases in preload and stroke volume develop during exercise, the increment in LV filling pressure is so great that the relation between LV stroke work and pulmonary wedge pressure is abnormal or frankly depressed.[7]

In morbidly obese subjects with hypoventilation syndrome, hypoxemia, and respiratory acidosis, pulmonary vasoconstriction may develop with a diastolic pressure gradient across the pulmonary vascular bed, thus, further elevating pulmonary artery and RV end-diastolic pressures above levels secondary to LV dysfunction alone.[4]

Hemodynamics in Obese Hypertensives

The presence of hypertension in markedly obese subjects (RBW 164.5% ± 2.7%) is associated with a lesser total and central blood volume and somewhat higher systemic vascular resistance, than that in normotensive obese subjects of comparable RBW.[10] However, elevation of cardiac output and stroke volume is approximately the same in both groups, and systemic vascular resistance with obesity hypertension is significantly less than that in lean hypertensives. Systemic vascular resistance may be within a normal range in obese hypertensives because of comparable increments in pressure and flow.[5,14] LV stroke work is higher in hypertensive than normotensive obese subjects, and may be considerably (60%) higher than in lean hypertensives because of the additional effect of increased LV preload and stroke volume.[10,22] Since myocardial hypertrophy tends to normalize LV wall tension in the setting of increased preload and end-diastolic dimension, the ratio of chamber radius to ventricular wall thickness (an index of wall stress) tends to remain in a normal range.[22] With marked obesity (RBW 174%), these increases in LV wall thickness and diastolic dimension are present both with and without hypertension.[22] In the absence of frank LV failure, the cardiac output response during exercise is within a normal range.[2,3] Elevation of LV diastolic and pulmonary wedge pressures in markedly obese hypertensives, at rest or during exercise, is comparable to, or slightly higher than, that of normotensive subjects with similar degrees of obesity.[2-5]

Hemodynamics in Obese Subjects with Congestive Heart Failure

Serial hemodynamic study of a normotensive morbidly obese subject presenting with congestive heart failure (CHF) has been reported by Kaltman and Goldring.[4] In this case, initial studies with failure and following weight reduction demonstrated increments in cardiac index and exercise factor (increment in cardiac output per 100 mL increase in body oxygen consumption) on weight loss, together with decrements in body oxygen consumption, arteriovenous oxygen content difference, LV and RV end-diastolic pressures, and central blood volume. On weight regain, cardiac index fell and ventricular filling pressures rose in conjunction with increased central blood volume. A second bout of weight reduction was accompanied by improvement in these parameters. The extent to which variations in ventricular function conditioned these hemodynamic findings is not clear, but in contrast to the findings in obese subjects without failure (vide infra) cardiac output rose with weight reduction.

In a cross-sectional study of 43 obese (BMI > 35 kg/m²) patients presenting with CHF, 67% had only myocardial hypertrophy on endomyocardial biopsy, Kasper and colleagues[23] found higher cardiac output but equally lowered cardiac indices as compared with lean subjects in congestive failure. Obese subjects also had higher pulmonary wedge, pulmonary artery, and right atrial mean pressures than did lean subjects. While these findings may characterize obesity cardiomyopathy, the range of body weights included subjects less than 225 lbs, and half of the subjects studied were in the BMI range of 35 to 40 kg/m^2, which raised the question of whether a large segment of those studied actually represented a group with "primary" idiopathic dilated cardiomyopathy who happened to be obese. Unfortunately, no selective data on those with BMI greater than 40 kg/m^2 are presented. However, the finding of hypertrophy on endomyocardial biopsy in 67% of cases was the same as that previously reported at necropsy in morbidly obese subjects.[24, 25]

Hemodynamic Effects of Weight Loss in Obese Subjects

The hemodynamic changes with weight loss in obese subjects, which reflected the quantitative degree of which adipose tissue metabolic demand and blood flow condition the overall circulatory state. In morbidly obese subjects who experience considerable weight reduction with gastric or other surgical procedures, these changes may be quite significant. The decrement in body oxygen consumption at rest with weight loss, which reflects the diminished metabolic demand of lesser adipose tissue in morbidly obese subjects, was 1.19 mL/min per kilogram in one study[14] and 1.35 in a second study,[27] in which the decrements in body weight averaged 53 and 58 kg. These decreases in body oxygen consumption were accompanied by decrements in circulating blood volume averaging 31 mL/kg weight loss in the first study and 17 in the second study. Arteriovenous oxygen difference at rest fell in both studies, which reflected a lesser oxygen extraction as adipose tissue volume fell. Reduced blood flow to adipose tissue resulted in lesser cardiac output at rest, which averaged 32 mL/min per kilogram weight loss in the first study and 24 in the second study. These decrements in blood volume averaged 1.65 and 1.0 L, and those in cardiac output 1.7 and 1.4 L/min, because of the large weight losses. In both studies, the percentage decrement in cardiac output with weight loss corresponded to the percentage decrement in blood volume. Mean brachial artery pressure at rest fell in both studies to 102 to 87 mm Hg and 102 to 93 mm Hg. There is little change in calculated systemic vascular resistance (Figure 2).[14] Modest decrements in mean

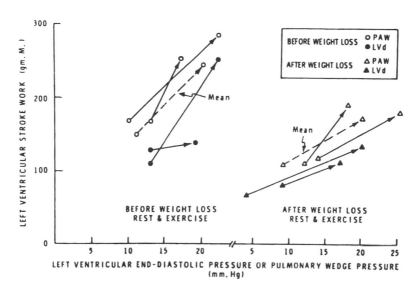

Figure 2. Effect of weight loss on systemic vascular resistance in severely obese subjects. Weight loss produces little change in systemic vascular resistance. The **closed circles** represent systemic vascular resistance before weight loss and **open circles** represent systemic vascular resistance after weight loss. The **dashed line** denotes the change in mean values induced by weight loss. (Reproduced from Reference 14 with permission.)

pulmonary artery pressure at rest were observed (19 to 15 mm Hg, and 20 to 16 mm Hg), but no significant change occurred in pulmonary wedge or LV diastolic pressure.

Oxygen uptake during exercise at comparable external workload is less following weight loss, as is the arteriovenous oxygen difference.[26] Stroke volume tends to be lower, which reflects a lower blood volume,[26] while heart rate may change little,[26] or fall,[7] at comparable external work loads. Increment in cardiac output per 100 mL increment in body oxygen consumption with exercise (exercise factor) increases.[4,14,26] Pulmonary artery pressures rise to a lesser degree during exercise following weight loss, but are still abnormally elevated.[14,26] Significant elevation of pulmonary wedge and LV diastolic pressures during exercise persist unchanged, though LV stroke work falls (Figure 3).[14,26] Thus, abnormal LV chamber compliance apparently persists for as long as 2 to 3 years after weight reduction despite diminution in LV mass.

In 12 hypertensive subjects with moderately severe obesity (RBW 164% ± 6% experiencing a mean weight loss of 10 kg (96 ± 4 to 86 ± 4 kg), hemodynamic changes following weight loss were quite similar to

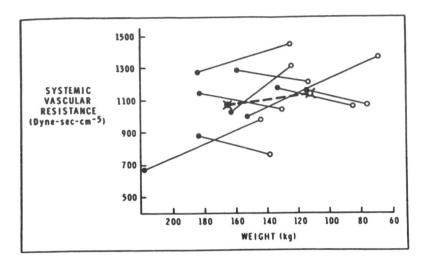

Figure 3. Effect of weight loss on pulmonary wedge pressure or left ventricular (LV) end-diastolic pressure and LV stroke work in severely obese patients. Pulmonary wedge pressure and LV end-diastolic pressure persisted unchanged while LV stroke work fell following weight loss. (Reproduced from Reference 14 with permission.)

those found in normotensive obese subjects.[27] A 10 mm Hg fall in mean systemic arterial pressure was accompanied by decrements in total blood volume, cardiac output, LV stroke work, and resting heart rate, with no significant change in stroke volume and total peripheral resistance. No change was found in renal and splanchnic blood flow or mean LV ejection rate.

Summary and Conclusions

Increments in resting body oxygen consumption and total blood volume parallel the total fat mass increments in obese subjects. Cardiac output, as measured using the Fick method, thermodilution, radionuclide, or echocardiographic methods correlate with indices of obesity, such as BMI and RBW, and may be double that at ideal weight in morbidly obese subjects. Resting heart rate changes little, so that cardiac stroke volume and work are increased. In contrast, central obesity is characterized by higher peripheral vascular resistance and lower cardiac output. Although splanchnic blood may be increased, the increment in cardiac output with obesity is largely distributed to adipose tissue. Cardiac output response to moderate exercise levels are within a normal range, but with higher exercise levels (5 METS), or in the setting of congestive failure, it is subnormal. Ventricular filling pressures in morbidly obese subjects (high normal or elevated at rest) rise to abnormal levels during exercise. With the obesity hypoventilation syndrome, pulmonary vascular resistance is increased, causing the need for further elevation of pulmonary artery pressure.

Relations among body weight, blood volume, and cardiac output in hypertensive obese subjects are similar to those in obese normotensive. Systemic vascular resistance is lower than in lean hypertensives, and may be normal because of comparable increments in pressure and flow. Elevation of LV diastolic and pulmonary wedge pressures at rest and during exercise may be somewhat greater than that of normotensive obese subjects at comparable RBW and BMI.

Obese subjects with cardiomyopathy who develop CHF tend to have higher cardiac output and ventricular filling pressures than lean subjects with dilated cardiomyopathy. Cardiac output at rest, and output response to exercise, may rise with weight reduction.

Weight loss of 55 kg over periods of 2 to 3 years, corresponding to 30% to 40% of total body weight in morbidly obese subjects, effects corresponding reductions in blood volume and cardiac output of 15% to 20%. Modest decreases in pulmonary wedge, pulmonary arterial, and LV diastolic pressures may be observed at rest, but they usually do not completely normalize. Cardiac output response to exercise improves, but intracardiac and pulmonary artery pressures rise abnormally. Pulmonary wedge and LV diastolic pressures rise with exercise to the same levels as those before weight loss, which is compatible with persistently diminished LV chamber compliance despite reduction in LV mass.

A weight loss of 10 kg in hypertensive subjects with moderately severe obesity may be accompanied by a reduction of 10 mm Hg in mean systemic arterial pressure, and hemodynamic alterations similar to those found in normotensive subjects.

References

1. Alexander JK, Dennis EW, Smith WG, et al: Blood volume, cardiac output and distribution of systemic blood flow in extreme obesity. *Cardiovasc Res Center Bull* 1:39–44, 1962.
2. Alexander JK: Obesity and cardiac performance. *Am J Cardiol* 14:860–865, 1964.
3. Backman L, Freyschuss U, Hallberg I, et al: Cardiovascular function in extreme obesity. *Acta Med Scand* 193:437–446, 1973.

4. Kaltman AJ, Goldring RM: Role of circulatory congestion in the cardiorespiratory failure of obesity. *Am J Med* 60:645–653, 1976.
5. DeDivitiis O, Fazio S, Petitto M, et al: Obesity and cardiac function. *Circulation* 64:477–482, 1981.
6. Agarwal N, Shibitani K, San Filippo JA, et al: Hemodynamic and respiratory changes in surgery of the morbidly obese. *Surgery* 92:226–235, 1982.
7. Alaud-din A, Meterissian S, Lisbona R, et al: Assessment of cardiac function in patients who were morbidly obese. *Surgery* 108:809–820, 1990.
8. Tucker GR, Alexander JK: Estimation of the body surface area of extremely obese human subjects. *J Appl Physiol* 15:781–784, 1960.
9. Messerli FH, Christie B, DeCarvalho JGR, et al: Obesity and essential hypertension. Hemodynamics, intravascular volume, sodium excretion and plasma renin activity. *Arch Intern Med* 141:81–85, 1981.
10. Messerli FH, Ventura HD, Reisin E et al: Borderline hypertension and obesity: Two prehypertensive states with elevated cardiac output. *Circulation* 66:55–60, 1982.
11. Merlino G, Scaglione R, Corrao E, et al: Association between reduced lymphocyte beta-adrenergic receptors and left ventricular dysfunction in young obese subjects. *Int J Obes* 18:699–703, 1994.
12. Nakajima T, Fujoka S, Tokagawa R, et al: Non-invasive study of left ventricular performance in obese patients: Influence of duration of obesity. *Circulation* 71:481–486, 1085.
13. Stoddard MF, Tseudo K, Thomas B, et al: The influence of obesity on left ventricular filling and systolic function. *Am Heart J* 124:694–699, 1992.
14. Alexander JK, Peterson KL: Cardiovascular effects of weight reduction. *Circulation* 45:310–318, 1972.
15. Jern S, Bergbrant A, Bjorntorp P, et al: Relation of central hemodynamics to obesity and body fat distribution. *Hypertension* 19:520–527, 1992.
16. Merlino G, Scaglione R, Paterna S, et al: Lymphocyte beta-adrenergic receptors in young subjects with peripheral or central obesity: Relationship with central hemodynamics and left ventricular function. *Eur Heart J* 15:786–792, 1994.
17. Smith WG, Alexander JK. Cerebral hemodynamics and oxygen utilization in extreme obesity. *Clin Sci* 20:33–39, 1960.
18. Kety SS, Schmidt CF: The nitrous oxide method for the quantitative determination of CBF in man: Theory, procedure and normal values. *J Clin Invest* 27:476–483, 1948.
19. Bradley SE, Ingelfinger FJ, Bradley GP, et al: Estimation of hepatic blood flow in man. *J Clin Invest* 24:890–897, 1945.
20. Messerli FH, Sundgaard-Reise K, Reisin E, et al: Disparate cardiovascular effects of obesity and arterial hypertension. *Am J Med* 74:808–812, 1983.
21. Nielsen SL: Measurement of blood flow in adipose tissue from the washout of xenon-133 after atraumatic labeling. *Acta Physiol Scand* 84(Suppl 2):187–196, 1972.
22. Messerli FH, Sungaard-Riise K, Reisin ED, et al: Dimorphic cardiac adaptation to obesity and arterial hypertension. *Ann Intern Med* 99:767–761, 1983.
23. Kasper EK, Hruban RH, Baughman KL: Cardiomyopathy of obesity: A

clinical pathologic evaluation of 43 obese patients with heart failure. *Am J Cardiol* 70:921–924, 1992.

24. Alexander JK: Obesity and the heart. *Curr Prob Cardiol* 5(3):6–41, 1980.
25. Warnes CA, Roberts WC: The heart in massive (more than 300 pounds or 136 kilograms) obesity: Analysis of 12 patients studied at necropsy. *Am J Cardiol* 54:1087–1091, 1984.
26. Backman L, Freyschuss U, Hallbert D, et al: Reversibility of cardiovascular changes in extreme obesity. Effects of weight reduction through jejeunoileostomy. *Acta Med Scand* 205:367–373, 1979.
27. Reisin E, Frohlich ED, Messerli FH, et al: Cardiovascular changes after weight loss in obesity hypertension. *Ann Intern Med* 98:315–319, 1983.
28. Alexander JK: The cardiomyopathy of obesity. *Prog Cardiovasc Dis* 27:325–344, 1984.
29. Alexander, JK: Cardiac effects of weight reduction in obesity hypertension. In Messerli FH, (ed) *The Heart and Hypertension.* Yorke Medical Books, New York, 1987, pp. 427–433.

Chapter 5

Obesity and Ventricular Function in Man
Diastolic Function

Simon Chakko, MD
Martin A. Alpert, MD
James K. Alexander, MD

Early studies of left ventricular (LV) diastolic function in obesity used cardiac catheterization as a diagnostic probe. Such studies were, by necessity, small.[1-3] Noninvasive techniques, such as Doppler echocardiography and radionuclide left ventriculography, have enabled us to study LV diastolic function in larger and more diverse populations. This chapter provides a review and analysis of studies assessing LV diastolic function in obesity at rest, during exercise, and following weight loss.

Evaluation of LV Diastolic Function

Diastole is a complex and active phenomenon which is energy dependent. It consists of four phases: isovolumic relaxation, rapid filling, diastasis, and atrial filling.[4] There is no currently available method that can completely and readily assess LV diastolic function.[5] Measures of diastolic function may be altered by changes in preload or afterload. Despite these limitations, evaluation of LV diastolic function is of great interest since in most disease states diastolic dysfunction precedes the onset of systolic dysfunction. As many as one-third of patients with con-

From: Alpert MA, and Alexander JK, (eds). *The Heart and Lung in Obesity*. Armonk, NY: Futura Publishing Company, Inc., © 1998.

gestive heart failure (CHF) have normal LV systolic function, and heart failure is attributable to diastolic dysfunction.[6] Before discussing the LV diastolic filling abnormalities seen in obesity, we will briefly describe the methods used to evaluate LV diastolic function.

Diastolic function may be evaluated by assessing the three diastolic properties (i.e., myocardial relaxation, ventricular compliance and diastolic filling).[4] Relaxation can be examined by measuring the exponential isovolumic LV pressure decline ($-Dp/dt$) during the isovolumic relaxation phases using high-fidelity, manometer-tipped catheters. Isovolumic relaxation time can be determined noninvasively by measuring the interval between aortic valve closure and mitral valve opening using Doppler echocardiography or a combination of phonocardiography and echocardiography. Normal isovolumic relaxation time ranges from 69 to 76 ms. It is prolonged by abnormal relaxation and shortened by elevated left atrial pressure.[5,7] Compliance or distensibility of the LV is assessed by measuring the relationship of ventricular diastolic pressure to ventricular volume in the cardiac catheterization laboratory.[4] A less compliant ventricle will have a higher than expected pressure at a given volume. Elevated LV end-diastolic pressure in the presence of normal systolic function usually indicates decreased compliance.[6]

LV filling can be evaluated by contrast ventriculography or by using noninvasive techniques such as Doppler echocardiography or radionuclide ventriculography. Recent studies have increasingly used noninvasive measures of LV filling to evaluate diastolic function. Filling rates can be measured either from a digitized echocardiogram or radionuclide ventriculogram. A continuous plot of LV dimension versus time is generated and peak filling rate is measured. Doppler echocardiography measures the flow across the mitral valve, which is dependent on the pressure difference between the LV and the left atrium that in turn is dependent on ventricular relaxation, compliance, and loading conditions. The transmitral Doppler E wave is the early filling velocity and the transmitral Doppler A wave is the atrial filling velocity (Figure 1). The ratio of E/A velocities is a measure of the role of atrial contribution to diastolic LV filling. The rate of decline in early filling velocity can be measured by the deceleration time, which is the time from peak E wave velocity to an extrapolation of the velocity to baseline (Figure 1). When myocardial relaxation is abnormal, a decrease in peak E wave velocity and E/A ratio occur and prolongation of deceleration and isovolumic relaxation times are observed (Figure 2). In the presence of improved LV compliance opposite changes occur: the E wave velocity and E/A ratio increase, deceleration and isovolumic relaxation times

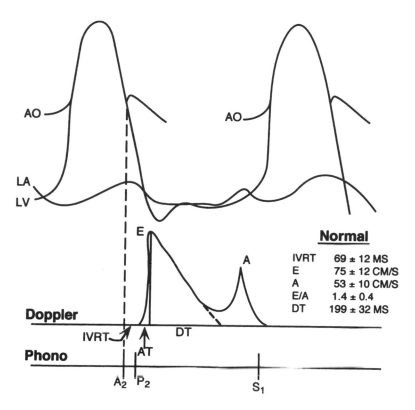

Figure 1. Relation of transmitral Doppler flow to left ventricular pressure (LV), left atrial pressure (LA), aortic pressure (AO), and to the heart sounds. Normal values for diastolic flow indices are shown in the **lower right.** A = transmitral Doppler A wave velocity; AT = acceleration time; A_2 and P_2 = aortic and pulmonic components of the second heart sound; DT = transmitral Doppler E wave and deceleration time; E = transmitral Doppler E wave velocity; E/A = E/A ratio; IVRT = isovolumic relaxation time; s_1 = first heart sound.

shorten, and A wave velocity decreases.[7] Increase in preload (elevation of left atrial pressure) results in changes similar to those seen with impaired compliance. Thus, impaired myocardial relaxation and elevated left atrial pressure lead to opposite changes. When left atrial pressure becomes elevated in the presence of impaired myocardial relaxation, the filling pattern may appear normal and is described as a "pseudo-normalized pattern." This pattern can be distinguished from a truly normal pattern by evaluation pulmonary venous flow that will show exaggerated flow reversal during atrial contraction if ventricular relaxation is impaired.

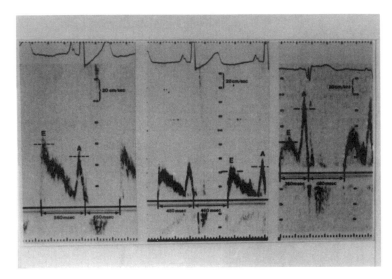

Figure 2. Normal and abnormal transmitral Doppler flow patterns. The tracing on the **left** shows normal transmitral pulse wave Doppler flow. Note that E (early filling) wave velocity exceeds A (late filling) wave velocity. The transmitral wave Doppler tracing in the **center** was obtained from a patient with impaired left ventricular (LV) diastolic filling. Note decreased E wave velocity and normal A wave velocity such that A wave velocity slightly exceeds E wave velocity. The tracing at the **far right** shows more severe impairment of LV diastolic filling with marked depression of E wave velocity, enhancement of A wave velocity, and reversal of the normal E/A wave flow relations. (From Hagan AD, DeMaria AN: *Clinical Applications of Two-Dimensional Echocardiography and Cardiac Doppler.* Little Brown and Co., Boston, 1989, p. 250.)

LV Filling Pressure at Rest and During Exercise

The fact that extremely obese patients may develop systemic and pulmonary vascular congestion in the absence of systolic dysfunction was well documented many years ago.[8] Alexander et al.[1] performed cardiac catheterization and obtained hemodynamic data at rest and during exercise in 40 obese subjects. Cardiac output was increased with a mean stroke volume of 100 mL. In 25% of cases pulmonary artery pressures were normal at rest and exercise and in another 25% pulmonary hypertension was present at rest and exercise; in the remaining 50% pulmonary hypertension was present during exercise only. Since pulmonary capillary wedge pressure was invariably elevated when pulmonary hypertension was present, elevation of LV filling pressure was determined to be the underlying cause of pulmonary hypertension. Increased cardiac workload at exercise was believed to cause myocardial insufficiency.

Backman et al.[2] obtained hemodynamic data at rest and exercise in 19 normotensive obese subjects (mainly women) whose body weight ranged from 108 to 172 kg. Mean cardiac output was 8.2 ± 1.7 L/min at rest and increased to 17.8 ± 2.9 L/min during exercise. The pulmonary capillary wedge pressure increased from 12 ± 3.6 mm Hg at rest to 21 ± 6.9 mm Hg with exercise. These investigators postulated that since the majority of the patients with elevated filling pressures did not have signs of clinical heart failure; impaired compliance of the LV was the cause of elevated filling pressures.

Kaltman and Goldring[3] also reported increased cardiac output and an abnormal exercise-induced elevation of mean LV end-diastolic pressure (12 to 30 mm Hg) in 19 obese patients. In addition, they also noted that there was a marked increase in mean LV end-diastolic pressure from 12 to 20 mm Hg with passive leg raising. These hemodynamic findings suggest that decreased LV compliance and increased blood volume are present in obese patients.

LV Diastolic Filling at Rest in Obese and Lean Patients

Although interpretable echocardiographic and cardiac Doppler studies may be technically difficult to obtain in the presence of obesity,[9] there is an increasing body of information derived from these techniques that provides a comparison of LV diastolic filling in obese and lean persons. Table 1 summarizes the results of six of these studies. Lavie et al.[10] reported significantly lower mean atrial emptying index in moderately obese patients than in lean controls matched for age, gender, and blood pressure. A similar relation was noted for obese and lean hypertensive patients, except that mean left atrial emptying index was lower in both subgroups than in normotensive patients.[11] Chakko and colleagues[11] compared Doppler diastolic filling patterns of normotensive obese and hypertensive lean patients with those of normal controls. Normotensive obese patients had eccentric LV hypertrophy, while hypertensive lean patients had concentric LV hypertrophy. The mean transmitral E/A ratio was significantly lower, the transmitral E wave deceleration half-time was significantly longer, and the peak filling rate was significantly less in obese patients than in controls. Similar relations were noted for obese and lean hypertensive patients. Obesity causes an increase in intravascular volume and filling pressures,[3,12] which would tend to mask the

Table 1
Comparative LV Diastolic Filling in Normotensive Obese and Lean Patients

Variable	Lavie et al[10]	Chakko et al[11]	Grossman et al[12]	Stoddard et al[13]	Wikstrand et al[14]	Ku et al[15]	Zarich et al[16]
Number	12 patients	21 patients; Obese 11 Lean 10	26 patients; Obese 13 Lean 13	48 patients; Obese 24 Lean 24	42 patients; Obese: 22 Lean: 20	60 patients; Obese 30 Lean 30	37 patients; Obese 21 Lean 16
Gender (F/M)	Obese: 2/10 Lean: 3/9	—	5/8 in both groups	—	Obese: 22/0 Lean: 20/0	15/15 in both groups	Obese: 13/3 Lean: Not provided
Mean age (years)	Obese 34 ± 2 Lean: 33 ± 3	Obese: 52 ± 14 Lean: 53 ± 13	Obese: 44 ± 4 Lean: 45 ± 3	34 ± 1	39.8	20 ± 1 in both groups	Obese: 38 Lean: Not provided
Severity of obesity							
BMI		30 kg/m²	>26, <35 kg/m²		25 kg/m²<40	25 kg/m²	—
% OW	>150%	—		>20%	—	—	128%
Modality used to assess LV diastolic filling	Echocardiography	Doppler echocardiography	Doppler echocardiography	Doppler echocardiography	Echocardiography	Doppler echocardiography	Doppler echocardiography
Transmitral Doppler E/A ratio							
Obese	—	1.0 ± 0.30	—	1.58 ± 0.53	—	0.6 ± 0.1*	1.16 ± 0.26
Lean	—	1.32 ± 0.21	—	1.54 ± 0.53	—	0.5 ± 0.20	1.66 ± 0.30
p	—	<0.05	—	N.S.	—	<0.01	<0.001
Transmitral E wave deceleration time (m/s)							
Obese	—	108 ± 9	—	—	—	—	—
Lean	—	86 ± 15	—	—	—	—	—
p	—	<0.05	—	—	—	—	—
Peak filling rate							
Obese	—	4.08 ± 0.65 sV/sec	8.2 ± 0.5				

Lean	—	4.96 ± 0.88 sV/sec	9.5 ± 0.3	—	—	—	—
p	—	<0.05	<0.04	—	—	—	—
Normalized peak filling rate (cm/s)							
Obese	—	—	2.2 ± 0.1	—	—	—	—
Lean	—	—	2.7 ± 0.1	—	—	—	—
p	—	—	<0.03	—	—	—	—
Isovolumic relaxation time (ms)							
Obese	—	—	—	84 ± 17	—	—	—
Lean	—	—	—	57 ± 13	—	—	—
p	—	—	—	<0.0001	—	—	—
% atrial contribution to LV filling							
Obese	—	—	—	—	—	—	36 ± 7
Lean	—	—	—	—	—	—	27 ± 4
p	—	—	—	—	—	—	<0.001
Left atrial emptying index (units)							
Obese	0.694 ± 0.06	—	—	—	—	—	—
Lean	0.855 ± 0.06	—	—	—	—	—	—
p	<0.01	—	—	—	—	—	—
LV relaxation time(s)							
Obese	—	—	—	—	107 ± 11	—	—
Lean	—	—	—	—	100 ± 6	—	—
p	—	—	—	—	<0.05	—	—

F = female; M = male; LV = left ventricular; OW = overweight; BMI = body mass index; * = A/E ratio rather than E/A ratio. All data are expressed as mean values ± 1 standard deviation.

Doppler-derived abnormalities of diastolic filling.[2,4] It is interesting that an abnormal filling pattern was seen despite the hemodynamics being unfavorable for its detection. Grossman et al.[13] studied the LV filling of mildly to moderately normotensive obese and normotensive lean patients. Mean peak filling rate and mean normalized peak filling rate in obese normotensive patients were significantly lower (more impaired) than in lean normotensive patients. There were no significant differences in duration of rapid filling between obese and lean normotensive patients. Similar relations were noted for obese and lean hypertensive patients except that diastolic filling was more impaired at baseline. Stoddard et al.[14] studied asymptomatic variably obese volunteers and compared them to age-matched normal lean controls. The obese subjects had a significantly longer mean isovolumic relaxation time than controls, probably due to abnormal myocardial relaxation. This is an interesting finding since increased blood volume, commonly found in obese subjects, tends to shortens the isovolumic relaxation time. In contrast to the other studies discussed, the ratio of transmitral E/A velocities was not significantly different in the obese subjects in this study, which may be explained by the lesser degree of LV hypertrophy.[14] Prolonged isovolumic relaxation time has also been noted in a study by Wikstrand and colleagues[15] that included only obese females. Ku et al.[16] studied mildly to moderately obese and lean patients. The mean transmitral A/E ratio in lean patients was significantly lower (less impaired) than that of the mean transmitral A/E ratio in obese patients. Mean late diastolic flow time and integral were significantly greater/longer (more impaired) in obese than in lean patients. Zarich and colleagues[17] studied normotensive severely obese patients and matched normotensive lean controls. The mean transmitral Doppler E/A ratio was significantly lower in obese than in lean subjects, and the mean percentage of atrial contribution to filling was significantly lower in lean than in obese patients. It is clear that obesity leads to abnormal LV relaxation and greater dependence on atrial contraction for ventricular filling. Many studies that evaluated diastolic function in hypertension may have overlooked the effect of obesity on diastolic filling.[18]

Factors Influencing LV Diastolic Function in the Obese

Factors influencing diastolic filling in the obese have been identified and include severity of obesity, increased LV mass, adverse alterations in LV loading conditions, duration of obesity, and the presence or absence of CHF.[19–24] DeDivitiis and colleagues[19] showed that in asymptomatic normotensive and mildly hypertensive obese subjects with no evidence of cardiac disease, pulmonary capillary wedge pressure, and LV end-diastolic pressure correlated positively and significantly with body weight. Some of the studies discussed earlier have also evaluated the correlation between diastolic filling abnormalities and body weight.[11,13,14,16] In the study by Chakko et al.[11] deceleration of early filling velocity correlated positively and significantly with body mass index. Peak filling rate measured by radionuclide ventriculography or echocardiography correlated positively and significantly with body weight and LV mass.[13,16] Stoddard et al.[14] performed multiple regression analysis to determine the correlation between various clinical and echocardiographic variables and diastolic filling parameters. Percentage of ideal body weight was the most important predictor of peak early filling velocity and mean deceleration time of early filling. More recent studies have focused on the influence of the severity of obesity on diastolic function. Scaglione et al.[21] measured diastolic filling rates using radionuclide ventriculography in lean subjects and patients with mild (25 to 30 kg/m²), and moderate (>30 and <40 kg/m²) obesity. Mean peak filling rate was significantly lower in mild and moderately obese patients than in lean patients. Mean time to peak filling rate decreased in a stepwise fashion with the degree of obesity. In the obese patients, peak filling rate correlated significantly and negatively with body mass index. Multiple regression analysis indicated that peak filling rate correlated with body mass index, but not with mean blood pressure or LV ejection fraction.

Obesity, as measured by body mass index or mass/height ratio, is an important and independent determinant of LV mass.[22] The amount overweight correlates positively and significantly with LV mass. A significant negative correlation was reported by Grossman et al.[13] between body mass index or LV mass and diastolic filling parameters. Alpert et al.[23] evaluated 50 asymptomatic, normotensive, and morbidly obese subjects (80% women) with Doppler echocardiography. The percent overweight correlated positively and significantly with LV mass/height index and the transmitral E wave deceleration time, and correlated negatively and significantly with the transmitral E/A ratio (Figure 3). There was a significant negative correlation between LV mass/height index and both E wave velocity and E/A ratio (Figure 4). A significant positive correlation was noted between LV mass/height index and both A wave velocity and E wave deceleration time (Figure 4). It was also noted that diastolic filling became progressively impaired as LV internal dimension in diastole, systolic blood pressure, and LV end-

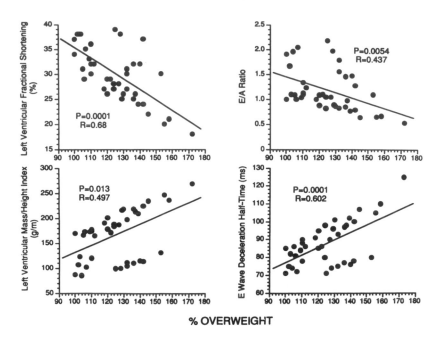

% OVERWEIGHT

Figure 3. Relation of percent overweight and left ventricular (LV) mass/height index and the transmitral Doppler E wave deceleration time and E/A ratio in morbidly obese patients. The percent overweight correlated positively and significantly with LV mass/height index and E wave deceleration time, and correlated negatively and significantly with the E/A ratio. (Reproduced from Reference 22 with permission.)

systolic wall stress increased (Figure 5). Thus, diastolic filling becomes progressively impaired as LV mass increases and as LV loading conditions that are known to predispose to LV hypertrophy (LV internal dimension in diastole, systolic blood pressure, and LV end-systolic wall stress) become more adverse. It is not clear whether the impairment in diastolic filling results from LV hypertrophy, per se, from alterations in LV loading conditions that predispose to LV hypertrophy, or both.

In a more recent study, Alpert and coworkers[24] evaluated the effect of duration of morbid obesity on LV mass, systolic function, and diastolic filling in 50 patients (80% women). The duration of morbid obesity correlated positively and significantly with the transmitral Doppler E wave deceleration time and negatively with the E/A ratio (Figure 6). In addition, there were positive and significant correlations between the duration of morbid obesity and the LV internal dimension in diastole, systolic blood pressure, LV end-systolic wall stress, and LV mass/

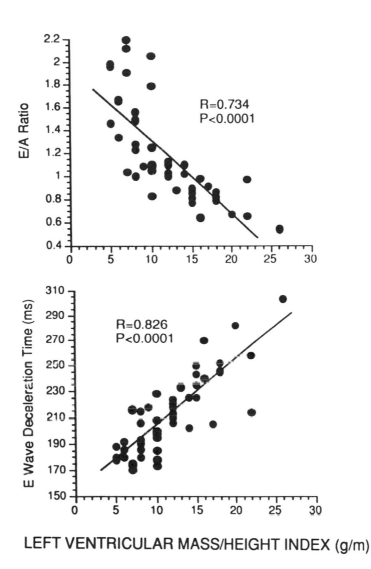

LEFT VENTRICULAR MASS/HEIGHT INDEX (g/m)

Figure 4. Relation of left ventricular (LV) mass/height index to transmitral Doppler E wave deceleration time and E/A ratio in morbidly obese patients. LV mass/height index correlated negatively and significantly with the E/A ratio, and correlated positively and significantly with the E wave deceleration time. (Reproduced from Reference 22 with permission.)

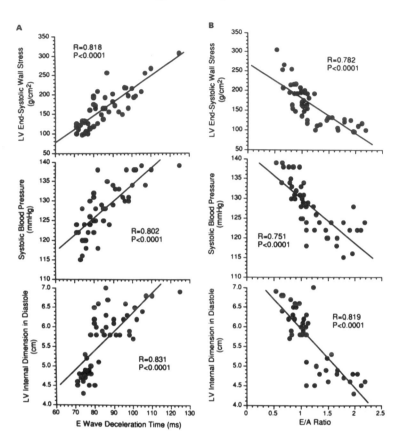

Figure 5. Relation of indices of left ventricular (LV) diastolic filling to the LV internal dimension in diastole, systolic blood pressure, and LV end-systolic wall stress in morbidly obese patients. Note the progressive increase in transmitral Doppler E wave deceleration time and the progressive decrease in E/A ratio (significantly greater impairment of diastolic filling) with increasing LV internal dimension in diastole, systolic blood pressure, and LV end-systolic wall stress. (Reproduced from Reference 22 with permission.)

height index (Figure 7). These data are supported by observations by Scaglione et al.,[20] which showed that peak filling rate correlated negatively and significantly with duration of mild to moderate obesity. Duration of morbid obesity was identified as a predictor of abnormal peak filling rate by multivariate analysis. Thus, longer duration of obesity is associated with higher LV mass, more adverse loading conditions, and greater impairment of LV diastolic filling.

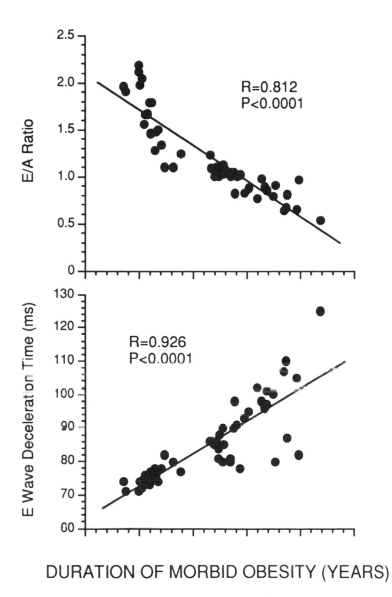

DURATION OF MORBID OBESITY (YEARS)

Figure 6. Relation of duration of morbid obesity to transmitral Doppler E wave deceleration time and E/A ratio. Duration of morbid obesity correlated positively and significantly with the E wave deceleration time and negatively and significantly with the E/A ratio. (Reproduced from *Am J Cardiol* 76:1194–1197, 1995 with permission.)

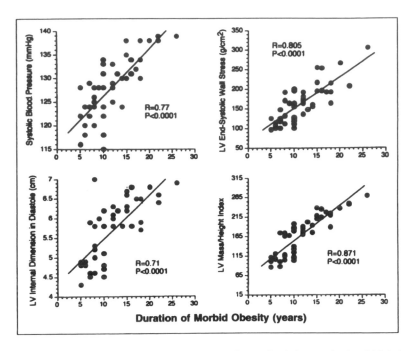

Figure 7. Relation of duration of morbid obesity to the left ventricular (LV) internal dimension in diastole, systolic blood pressure, and LV mass/height index. Duration of morbid obesity correlated positively and significantly with each of these variables. (Reproduced from *Am J Cardiol* 76:1194–1197, 1995 with permission.)

Alpert and coworkers[25] studied 74 morbidly obese patients (approximately 80% women) to compare LV diastolic filling in those with and without CHF. There were 24 patients with and 50 patients without CHF. The mean transmitral Doppler E wave deceleration time was significantly longer in patients with CHF (264 ± 34 ms) than in those without CHF (213 ± 30 ms). The mean transmitral Doppler E/A ratio was significantly lower in patients with CHF (0.79 ± 0.25) than in those without CHF (1.20 ± 0.43). Of note, the mean LV internal dimension in diastole, mean systolic blood pressure, mean LV end-systolic wall stress, mean LV mass/height index, and mean duration of morbid obesity were all significantly longer/higher/greater in patients with than in those without CHF. Thus, the greater impairment of LV diastolic filling in morbidly obese patients with than in those without CHF relates, at least in part, to longer duration of obesity, greater LV mass, and more adverse LV loading conditions.

Effect of Weight Loss on LV Diastolic Filling

Two studies have demonstrated that LV diastolic filling improves following substantial weight loss in obese individuals. Alpert and coworkers[26] studied 25 morbidly obese subjects (primarily women). The percent overweight decreased from 131% ± 17% prior to 38% ± 5% after vertical band gastroplasty. In patients with increased LV mass/height index, the mean transmitral Doppler E/A ratio increased significantly from 0.83 ± 0.16 to 1.20 ± 0.14. The mean transmitral Doppler E wave deceleration time decreased significantly from 247 ± 21 ms prior to 200 ± 19 ms following weight loss. These changes were accompanied by significant reductions in the mean LV internal dimension in diastole, mean systolic blood pressure, and mean LV end-systolic wall stress. Such changes were not noted in those with normal LV mass/height index. The magnitude of weight loss-induced decreases in LV mass/height index, LV internal dimension in diastole, systolic blood pressure, and LV end-systolic wall stress all correlated strongly with improvements in diastolic filling (Figures 8 and 9). Thus, weight loss-induced improvements in diastolic filling in morbidly obese subjects occur primarily and perhaps exclusively in those with increased LV mass and are associated with both a decrease in LV mass and improvement in LV loading conditions. In a subsequent study, Alpert and coworkers[24] reported that patients with longer durations of morbid obesity experienced greater improvement in LV diastolic filling following weight loss.

DasGupta et al.[26] studied diastolic filling before and after diet-induced weight loss (mean 10 kg) in 11 normotensive mildly to moderately obese subjects (mainly women). Diet-induced weight loss produced a significant decrease in mean peak filling rate from 2.71 ± 0.73 SV/sec before weight loss to 2.05 ± 0.59 SV/sec after weight loss. There were no significant changes in the mean time to peak filling rate or mean filling fraction during the first third of diastole. Mean filling fraction, but not mean peak filling rate or mean time, to peak filling rate was significantly lower in normotensive obese patients than in normals. There were no significant differences pre- and post-diet for any mean diastolic filling variable in 15 hypertensive patients.

In contrast to these studies, Reid and coworkers[27] reported no improvement in diastolic filling following weight loss in a small study of overweight subjects.

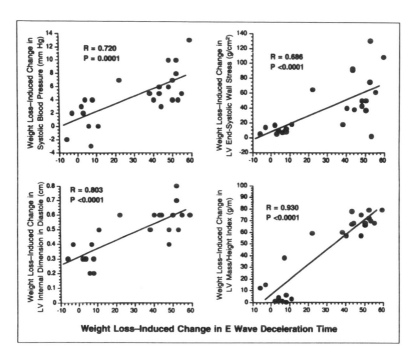

Figure 8. Relation of weight loss-induced changes in transmitral Doppler E wave deceleration time to the left ventricular (LV) internal dimension in diastole, systolic blood pressure, and LV end-systolic wall stress in morbidly obese patients. The magnitude of weight loss-induced change (decreases) in E wave deceleration time correlated significantly with the magnitude if weight loss-induced change in the LV internal dimension in diastole, systolic blood pressure, and LV end-systolic wall stress. (Reproduced from *Am J Cardiol* 76:1198–1201, 1995 with permission.)

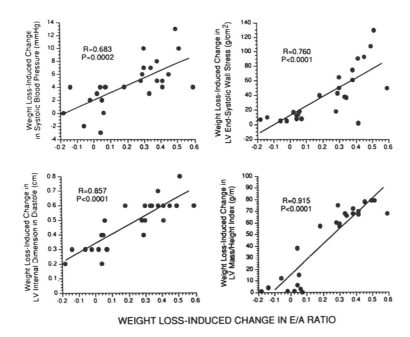

WEIGHT LOSS-INDUCED CHANGE IN E/A RATIO

Figure 9. Relation of weight loss-induced changes in transmitral E/A ratio to the left ventricular (LV) internal dimension in diastole, systolic blood pressure, and LV end-systolic wall stress in morbidly obese patients. The magnitude of increase in E/A ratio correlated positively and significantly with the magnitude of decrease in the LV internal dimension in diastole, systolic blood pressure, and LV end systolic wall stress. (Reproduced from *Am J Cardiol* 76:1198–1201, 1995 with permission.)

Summary and Conclusions

In summary, eccentric LV hypertrophy with obesity in association with unfavorable alterations in LV loading conditions leads to diastolic dysfunction. Diastolic filling abnormalities have been demonstrated by many investigators using cardiac catheterization, echocardiography, and radionuclide left ventriculography. The degree of diastolic dysfunction is related to the severity of obesity, duration of obesity, increased LV mass, and unfavorable alterations in LV loading conditions, and is more severe in those with CHF than in those without. Diastolic filling improves following weight reduction, particularly in those with LV hypertrophy. Such improvement occurs in association with regression of LV hypertrophy and improvement in LV loading conditions.

References

1. Alexander JK: Obesity and cardiac performance. *Am J Cardiol* 14:860–865, 1964.
2. Backman L, Freyschuss U, Hallberg D, et al: Cardiovascular function in extreme obesity. *Acta Med Scand* 193:437–446, 1973.
3. Kaltman AJ, Goldring RM: Role of circulatory congestion in cardiorespiratory failure of obesity. *Am J Med* 60:645–653, 1976.
4. Harizi RC, Bianco JA, Alpert JS: Diastolic function of the heart in clinical cardiology. *Arch Intern Med* 148:99–109, 1988.
5. Nishimura RA, Abel MD, Hatle LK, et al: Assessment of diastolic function of the heart: Background and current applications of Doppler echocardiography. Part I. Physiologic and pathophysiologic features. *Mayo Clin Proc* 64:71–81, 1989.
6. Bonow RO, Udelson JE: Left ventricular diastolic dysfunction as a cause of congestive heart failure. Mechanisms and management. *Ann Intern Med* 117:502–510, 1992.
7. Nishimura RA, Abel MD, Hatle LK, et al: Assessment of diastolic function of the heart: Background and current applications of Doppler echocardiography. Part II. Clinical studies. *Mayo Clin Proc* 64:181–204, 1989.
8. Alexander JK: The cardiomyopathy of obesity. *Prog Cardiovasc Dis* 27:325–334, 1985.
9. Alpert MA, Kelly DL: Value and limitations of echocardiography in the assessment of obese patients. *Echocardiography* 3:261–272, 1986.
10. Lavie CJ, Amodeo C, Ventura HO, et al: Left atrial abnormalities indicating diastolic ventricular dysfunction in cardiomyopathy of obesity. *Chest* 92:1042–1046, 1987.
11. Chakko S, Mayer M, Allison MD, et al: Abnormal left ventricular diastolic filling in eccentric left ventricular hypertrophy of obesity. *Am J Cardiol* 68:95–98, 1991.
12. Alpert MA, Hashimi MW: Obesity and the heart. *Am J Med Sci* 306:117–123, 1993.
13. Grossman E, Oren S, Messerli FH: Left ventricular filling in the systemic hypertension of obesity. *Am J Cardiol* 68:57–60, 1991.
14. Stoddard MF, Tseuda K, Thomas M, et al: The influence of obesity on left ventricular filling and systolic function. *Am Heart J* 124:694–699, 1992.
15. Wikstrand J, Pettersson P, Bjorntorp P: Body fat distribution and left ventricular morphology and function in obese females. *J Hypertens* 11:1259–1266, 1993.
16. Ku CS, Lin SL, Wang DJ, et al: Left ventricular filling in young normotensive obese adults. *Am J Cardiol* 73:613–615, 1994.
17. Zarich EW, Kowalchi GJ, Benotti PN, et al: Left ventricular filling abnormalities in asymptomatic morbid obesity. *Am J Cardiol* 68:377–381, 1991.
18. Egan B, Fitzpatrick A, Juni J, et al: Importance of overweight in studies of left ventricular hypertrophy and diastolic function in mild systemic hypertension. *Am J Cardiol* 64:752–755, 1989.
19. De Divitiis O, Fazio S, Petitto M, et al: Obesity and cardiac function. *Circulation* 64:477–482, 1981.
20. Scaglione R, Dichiara MA, Indovina R, et al: Left ventricular diastolic and

systolic function in normotensive obese subjects: Influence of degree and duration of obesity. *Eur Heart J* 13:138–142, 1992.

21. Hammond IW, Devereux RB, Alderman WH, et al: Relation of blood pressure and body build to left ventricular mass in normotensive and hypertensive employed adults. *J Am Coll Cardiol* 12:996–1004, 1988.

22. Alpert MA, Lambert CR, Terry BE, et al: Interrelationship of left ventricular mass, systolic function and diastolic filling in normotensive morbidly obese patients. *Int J Obes* 19:550–557, 1995.

23. Alpert MA, Lambert CR, Panayiotou H, et al: Relation of duration of morbid obesity to left ventricular mass, systolic function and diastolic filling and effect of weight loss. *Am J Cardiol* 76:1194–1197, 1995.

24. Alpert MA, Terry BE, Mulckar M, et al: Cardiac morphology and left ventricular function in normotensive morbidly obese patients with and without congestive heart failure and effect of weight loss. *Am J Cardiol,* in press.

25. DasGupta P, Ramhanmdany E, Brigden G, et al: Improvement of left ventricular function after rapid weight loss in obesity. *Eur Heart J* 13:1060–1066, 1992.

26. Alpert MA, Lambert CR, Terry BE, et al: Effect of weight loss on left ventricular diastolic filling in obesity. *Am J Cardiol* 76:1198–1201, 1995.

27. Reid CM, Dart AM, Dewar EM, et al: Interactions between the effects of exercise and weight loss on risk factors, cardiovascular hemodynamics and left ventricular structure in overweight subjects. *J Hypertension* 12:291–301, 1994.

Chapter 6

Obesity and Ventricular Function in Man

Systolic Function

Martin A. Alpert, MD
James K. Alexander, MD
Simon Chakko, MD

Left ventricular (LV) systolic function in obesity has been studied extensively. Right ventricular (RV) systolic function has received comparatively less attention. This chapter provides a review and analysis of studies assessing the effects of obesity on LV and RV systolic function at rest, during exercise, and following weight loss.

Assessment of LV Systolic Function

Systole is a complex, energy-dependent portion of the cardiac cycle that consists of four phases: isovolumic contraction, rapid ventricular ejection, reduced ventricular ejection, and protodiastole.[1] LV and RV systolic function are assessed most commonly using ejection phase indices.[2-4] Such indices are commonly measured in the clinical setting using contrast left ventriculography, echocardiography, radionuclide angiography, and systolic time intervals. These include left ventricular ejection fraction (LVEF), right ventricular ejection fraction (RVEF), left ventricular fractional shortening (LVFS), the mean velocity of LV circumferential fiber shortening (mean VcF), and the ratio of the

From: Alpert MA, and Alexander JK, (eds). *The Heart and Lung in Obesity.* Armonk, NY: Futura Publishing Company, Inc., © 1998.

pre-ejection period to the LVET. Angiographic and echocardiographic LVEF is defined by the following formula[2]:

$$\text{LVEF (\%)} = \frac{\text{LV End-Diastolic Volume} - \text{LV End-Systolic Volume}}{\text{LV End-Diastolic Volume}} \times 100$$

Radionuclide LVEF and RVEF are defined by the following formulae[3]:

$$\text{LVEF (\%)} = \frac{\text{LV Counts In Diastole} - \text{LV Counts In Systole}}{\text{LV Counts in Diastole}} \times 100$$

$$\text{RVEF (\%)} = \frac{\text{RV Counts In Diastole} - \text{RV Counts In Systole}}{\text{RV Counts in Diastole}} \times 100$$

LVFS is assessed using echocardiography and is defined by the following formula[4]:

$$\text{LVFS (\%)} = \frac{\text{LV Internal Dimension In Diastole} - \text{LV Internal Dimension In Systole}}{\text{LV Internal Dimension In Diastole}} \times 100$$

Mean VcF is assessed using echocardiographic or angiographic techniques and is expressed as circumferences per second (circ/sec). It is defined by the following formula[4]:

$$\text{Mean VcF (circ/sec)} = \frac{\text{LV Internal Dimension In Diastole} - \text{LV Internal Dimension In Systole}}{\text{LV Internal Dimension In Diastole} \times \text{LV Ejection Time}} \times 100$$

The pre-ejection period (PEP)/left ventricular ejection time ratio (LVET) is typically assessed using echocardiography or phonocardiography in combination with carotid pulse tracings.[4] The higher the ratio, the more LV systolic function is impaired.

It is important to emphasize that all of these ejection phase indices are load dependent. Each may be affected by changes in preload and afterload (unlike V_{max}) and are, therefore, not true indices of the inotropic state.

LV Systolic Function at Rest in Obese and Lean Patients

Studies assessing LV systolic function at rest in obese and lean patients have produced conflicting results. Table 1 summarizes the results of these studies. Investigators from Italy found that mean LVEF and mean LV ejection rate were significantly lower in moderately obese subjects than in either mildly obese or lean patients.[5] These investigators also reported significantly lower mean LVEF values in mildly to moderately centrally obese and peripherally obese patients than in lean controls (Table 1).[6] Lymphocyte β-adrenergic receptor density was significantly lower in obese than lean patients.[6] The precise cause of reduced lymphocyte β-adrenergic receptor density in those with LV systolic dysfunction is unclear. Moreover, it is uncertain whether myocardial β-adrenergic receptors were affected in the same way as lymphocyte β-adrenergic receptors. In contrast, several studies of normotensive[7-9] and hypertensive[9] adults have failed to identify a significant difference in LV systolic function between mildly to moderately obese and lean patients (Table 1). Similarly, a study of moderately obese children by Koehler et al.[10] showed no significant difference in LV systolic function between obese and lean groups (Table 1). Ventura et al.[11] reported a study of two groups of hypertensive patients with comparable mean LVEF values immediately after cardiac transplantation (64% ± 3% and 64% ± 2%, respectively). However, 1 year after cardiac transplantation, mean LVEF was significantly lower in those who gained weight (34% ± 4%), than in those who had not gained weight (57% ± 3%).

Factors Influencing Left Ventricular Systolic Function

Several factors have been identified that influence LV systolic function in obese patients. These include the severity of obesity, LV loading conditions and mass, duration of obesity, the presence or absence of congestive heart failure (CHF), and possibly hemostatic function.

Two studies have reported a correlation between severity of obesity and LV systolic function. In a study of 24 mildly to moderately obese patients, Stoddard et al.[8] reported a moderate yet significant, negative correlation between the percent of ideal body weight and LVEF, and a moderately, significant positive correlation between the percent over ideal

Table 1

Comparative Left Ventricular Systolic Function at Rest in Normotensive Obese and Lean Patients

Variable	Scaglione et al[5]	Merlino et al[6]	Veille et al[7]	Stoddard et al[8]	Messerli et al[9]	Koehler et al[10]
Number	27 patients OW: 10 ModOb: 7 Lean: 10	51 patients CentOb: 9 PeriOb: 22 Lean: 20	44 pregnant women Obese: 8 Lean: 36	48 patients Obese: 24 Lean: 24	34 patients Obese: 17 Lean: 17	61 children Obese: 41 Lean: 26
Gender (F/M)	OW: 5/5; ModOb: 4/3; Lean: 6/4	CentOb: 4/5; PeriOb: 11/11; Lean: 10/10	All women	Not provided	Obese: 7/10; Lean: 7/10	Not provided
Mean age (years)	OW: 40.2 ± 3.5; ModOb: 48.6 ± 2.1; Lean: 44.7 ± 2.2	CentOb: 36.0 ± 3.7; PeriOb: 36.3 ± 3.9; Lean: 36.9 ± 3.5	Obese: 35 ± 3; Lean: 27 ± 1	34 ± 1	34 ± 10	Not provided
Severity of obesity	OW: 25–30 kg·m²; ModOb: >30 <40 kg/m²	M: >30.5 kg·m² F: >27.3 kg·m²	≥150% of ideal body weight	>20% OW	>150% of ideal body weight	76 ± 10% OW
Modality used to assess LV systolic function	Echocardiography	RNV	Echocardiography	Echocardiography	Echocardiography	Echocardiography
LVEF (%) Obese	OW: 61.5 ± 2.1; ModOb: 57.5 ± 2.2	CentOb: 57.1 ± 4.6; PeriOb: 61.2 ± 4.0	—	59 ± 5	—	73 ± 12
Lean	65.0 ± 1.8	65.5 ± 4.0	—	58 ± 4	—	77 ± 5
P	<0.05 (lean vs. ModOb and OW)	<0.05 (lean vs. CentOb and PeriOb)	—	N.S.	—	N.S.

Mean Vcf (circ/sec)					
Obese	—	—	—	112.9 ± 24.9	1.40 ± 0.75
Lean	—	—	—	113.4 ± 18.2	1.49 ± 0.29
P	—	—	—	N.S.	N.S.
PEP/LVET ratio					
Obese	—	—	0.31 ± 0.06	—	—
Lean	—	—	0.27 ± 0.06	—	—
P	—	—	<0.02	—	—
LV Fractional shortening (%)					
Obese	41 ± 2	35 ± 8	—	—	—
Lean	38 ± 1	36 ± 6	—	—	—
P	N.S.	N.S.	—	—	—

F = female; M = male; LV = left ventricular; LVEF = left ventricular ejection fractional Mean Vcf = mean velocity of circumferential fiber shortening (circumferences/second); PEP/LVET = pre-ejection period to left ventricular ejection time ratio; OW = overweight; ModOb = moderately obese; CenOb = centrally obese; PeriOb = peripherally obese; RNV = radionuclide ventriculography.
Mean values are expressed as ± 1 standard deviation.

body weight and PEP/LVET. Alpert and coworkers[12] noted a moderate yet significant, negative correlation between the percent overweight and LVFS in 50 morbidly obese individuals (mainly women) (Figure 1).[12]

LV loading conditions and LV mass may also influence LV systolic function. In a study of 50 morbidly obese patients (mainly women), Alpert et al.[12] assessed the relation of LV systolic function and loading conditions. LVFS correlated negatively and significantly with the LV internal dimension in diastole, LV end-systolic wall stress, and systolic blood pressure (Figure 2). LVFS also correlated negatively and significantly with LV mass/height index (Figure 3). These findings extended those of a previous study by Alexander et al.,[13] which showed a positive correlation between LVFS and LV end-systolic stress in morbidly obese patients, and an early report of Alpert and coworkers,[14] which demonstrated the importance of LV loading conditions and LV mass in determining LV systolic function.

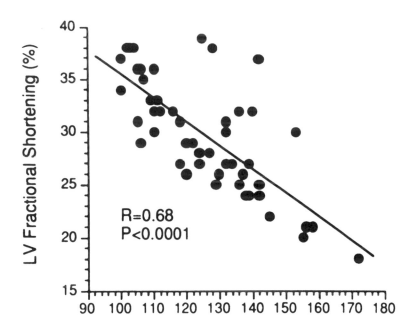

% Overweight

Figure 1. Relation of percent overweight to left ventricular fractional shortening (LVFS) in morbidly obese patients. LVFS correlates negatively and significantly with percentage overweight. (Reproduced from Reference 12 with permission.)

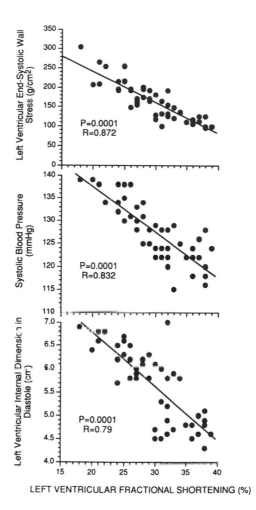

Figure 2. Relation of left ventricular fractional shortening (LVFS) to the left ventricular (LV) internal dimension in diastole, systolic blood pressure, and LV end-systolic wall stress in morbidly obese patients. LVFS correlates negatively and significantly with all of these variables. (Reproduced from Reference 12 with permission.)

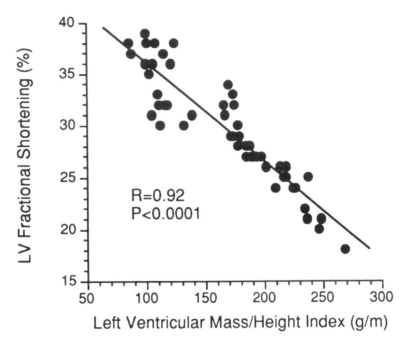

Figure 3. Relation of left ventricular (LV) mass/height index to left ventricular fractional shortening (LVFS) in morbidly obese patients. LVFS correlates negatively and significantly with LV mass/height index. (Reproduced from Reference 12 with permission.)

Duration of obesity may also be an important determinant of LV systolic function. In a study of 50 normotensive severely obese patients (80% women), there was a significant negative correlation between duration of morbid obesity and LVFS (Figure 4). However, duration of morbid obesity correlated significantly and positively with the LV internal dimension in diastole, systolic blood pressure, LV end-systolic wall stress, and LV mass/height index (Figure 5).[15] Thus, it was not possible to determine whether the apparent influence of duration of morbid obesity on LV systolic function was independent or due primarily to changes in LV loading conditions or mass. In contrast, Nakajima et al.[16] reported no significant differences in either mean VcF or LVFS between 18 normotensive moderately obese patients who were obese for 15 years or less and 17 normotensive moderately obese patients who were obese for greater than 15 years.

In a study of 24 normotensive morbidly obese patients with and 50 normotensive morbidly obese patients without CHF, Alpert et al.[17] re-

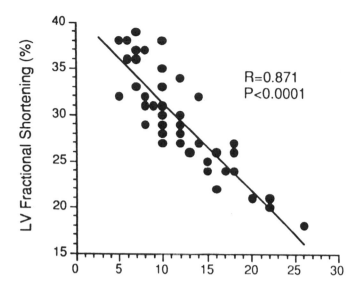

Figure 4. Relation of duration of morbid obesity to left ventricular fractional shortening (LVFS). LVFS correlates negatively and significantly with duration of morbid obesity. (Reproduced from *Am J Cardiol* 76:1194–1197, 1005 with permission.)

ported that mean LVFS was significantly lower in patients with (23% ± 5 %) than in those without CHF (29% ± 5 %). Mean duration of severe obesity, mean LV internal dimension in diastole, mean systolic blood pressure, and mean LV end-systolic wall stress were all significantly longer/larger/higher, and greater in severely obese patients with than those without CHF.[17] Thus, the greater impairment of LV systolic function in those with CHF than in those without relates, at least in part, to longer duration of severe obesity, increased LV mass, and more adverse LV loading conditions.

Licata et al.[18] assessed the relation of hemostatic function and echocardiographic LV systolic function in 19 obese and 20 lean individuals. Obesity was defined as body mass index $\geq$30.5 kg/m^2 in men and $\geq$27.3 kg/m^2 in women. There were significant negative correlations between LVEF and platelet activator inhibitor, tissue plasminogen activator 1, and fibrinogen. The reason for this association remains unclear.

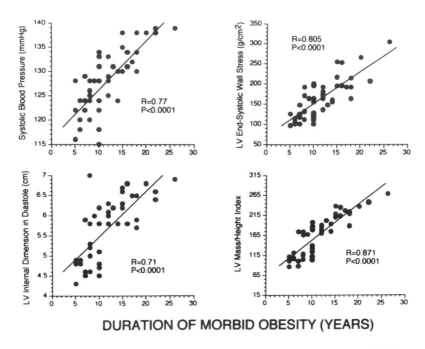

Figure 5. Relation of duration of morbid obesity to the left ventricular (LV) internal dimension in diastole, systolic blood pressure, and LV end-systolic wall stress. Duration of morbid obesity correlates positively and significantly with all of these variables. (Reproduced from *Am J Cardiol* 76:1194–1197, 1995 with permission.)

Effect of Exercise on Left and Right Ventricular Function

In normotensive lean individuals, increasing increments of exercise produce a progressive increase in LV systolic function. Four studies have explored the effect of exercise on LV systolic function in obese subjects. The results of these studies are summarized in Table 2. Licata et al.[19] demonstrated that exercise produces a significant increase in LVEF in mildly, but not moderately obese subjects. In mildly obese patients whose duration of obesity was less than 12 months, exercise produced a significant increase in LVEF. Such was not observed in those with moderate obesity for less than 120 months, or in either subgroup in subjects obese for ≥ 120 months. There was no correlation between resting LVEF and the exercise induced change in LVEF. Alaud-din et al.[20] found that exercise produced no significant change in mean LVEF in morbidly obese patients (Table 2). Alpert and colleagues[21] reported a

Table 2
Effect of Exercies on Left and Right Ventricular Systolic Function in Obese Patients

Variable	Licata et al[19] Mildly Obese	Licata et al[19] Moderately Obese	Alaud-din et al[20] Before Gastroplasty	Alaud-din et al[20] After Gastroplasty	Alpert et al[21] Normal LV Mass	Alpert et al[21] Increased LV Mass	Alpert et al[22] RVID <2.0 cm	Alpert et al[22] RVID ≥2.0 cm
Number	15	14	12		23		22	
Gender (F/M)	9/6	9/5	Not provided		18/5		17/5	
Mean age (years)	41.13 ± 2.64	43.78 ± 2.52	Not provided		37 ± 7		36 ± 8	
Severity of obesity	Mild	Moderate	Severe		Severe		Severe	
BMI	25–30 kg/m²	<40 kg/m²	49 ± 71 kg/m²	28 ± 7 kg/m²				
% OW	—	—			139 ± 12% OW		129 ± 16	
Modality used to measure LV systolic function	RNV	RNV	RNV		RNV		RNV	
Exercise Modality	Bicycle ergometry Symptom-limited		Bicycle ergometry		Bicycle ergometry Symptom-limited		Bicycle ergometry Symptom-limited	
Exercise End-Point(s)	72 ± 2 W	70 ± 2 W	25 and 50 W		40 W increments		40 W increments	
LVEF (%)								
Rest	60.4 ± 1.4	58.2 ± 1.2	48 ± 2.9	54.7 ± 2.8	54 ± 8	53 ± 10	—	—
Exercise	65.9 ± 1.2	59.8 ± 1.5	25 W 50.6 ± 3.1 / 50W 53.0 ± 3.1	59.3 ± 3.2 / 59.1 ± 2.9	66 ± 12	50 ± 12	—	—
P	<0.05	N.S.	N.S. (rest vs. 25 or 50 W)	N.S. (rest vs. 25 or 50 W)	<0.001	N.S.	—	—
RVEF (%)								
Rest	—		—		—		43 ± 10	
Exercise	—		—		—		58 ± 11	
P	—		—		—		<0.03	

F = female; M = male; BMI = body mass index; OW = overweight; LV = left ventricular; LVEF = left ventricular ejection fraction; RVEF = right ventricular ejection fraction; RVID = right ventricular internal dimension; RNV = radionuclide ventriculography; W = watts.
Mean values are expressed as ± 1 standard deviation.

significant exercise related increase in LVEF in severely obese patients with normal LV mass, but no significant change in LVEF in those with increased LV mass (Table 2). Of note, the mean LV radius to thickness ratio was substantially higher in patients with increased LV mass, which suggested that increased LV wall stress may have played a key role in determining LV systolic function and reserve. There was a significant negative correlation between LV mass and the exercise related change in LVEF (Figure 6).

In the only study on the effect of exercise on RV systolic function, Alpert and coworkers[22] showed that in morbidly obese patients RVEF increased significantly with exercise when the RV internal dimension was less than 2.0 cm. Exercise produced no significant change in severely obese subjects whose RV internal dimension was 2.0 cm or more. RV exercise response correlated negatively and significantly with the RV internal dimension.

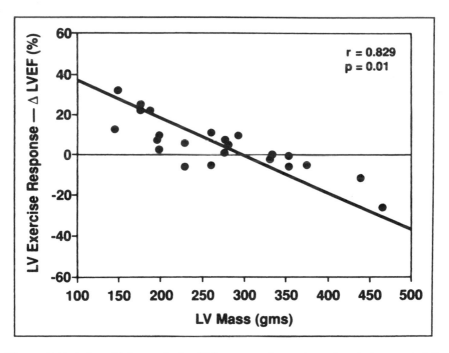

Figure 6. Relation of left ventricular (LV) mass and exercise-related changes in left ventricular ejection fraction (LVEF) in morbidly obese patients. Exercise-related changes in LVEF correlated negatively and significantly with LV mass. (Reproduced from *Am J Cardiol* 63:1478–1482, 1989 with permission.)

Effect of Weight Loss on LV Systolic Function

An increasing body of evidence suggests that weight loss may produce improvement in LV systolic function in the obese.[14, 23, 24] Such an improvement has occurred in mildly, moderately, and morbidly obese patients, and with a variety of weight reduction methods. Table 3 summarizes the results of studies addressing this issue.

Alpert et al.[14] studied 39 normotensive morbidly obese patients (mainly women) and noted that substantial weight loss from gastroplasty produced a significant increase in mean LVFS in those with depressed LVFS prior to weight loss (Table 3). This was accompanied by significant decreases in the mean LV internal dimension in diastole, mean systolic blood pressure, and mean LV end-systolic wall stress. This was not observed in morbidly obese patients with normal LV systolic function prior to weight loss (Table 3). In this study, there were significant positive correlations between the weight loss-related changes in LVFS and the pre-weight loss LV internal dimension in diastole, systolic blood pressure, and LV end-systolic wall stress. Pre-weight loss LVFS correlated negatively and significantly with the weight loss induced change in LVFS. Finally, there were significant negative correlations between the weight-loss related change in LVFS and weight loss-related changes in systolic blood pressure and LV end-systolic wall stress (Figure 7), but not the LV internal dimension in diastole.

Improvement in LV systolic function following weight loss has also been described by Wirth and Kröger[23] in moderately obese patients following dietary weight loss, but not from weight loss induced by a combination of diet plus exercise (Table 3). In contrast, DasGupta and colleagues[24] reported no significant change in LV systolic function following weight loss in mildly obese patients (Table 3).

Limited information is available concerning LV exercise response in the obese patient following weight loss. In the study by DasGupta and colleagues[24] of mildly obese patients, LVEF with exercise did not change significantly before weight loss, but increased significantly after weight loss. Alaudin-din and coworkers[20] reported small increments in LVEF following weight loss in 12 morbidly obese patients. These increases were not statistically significant, but may indicate a trend towards improvement in LV systolic function following weight loss in such individuals.[20]

The findings of these studies suggest that weight loss is capable of producing improvement in LV systolic function in moderately to se-

Table 3
Effect of Weight Loss on Left Ventricular Systolic Function in Obese Patients

Variable	Alpert et al[14] Normal LVFS (≥28%)	Alpert et al[14] Depressed LVSF (<28%)	Wirth et al[23] Diet Alone	Wirth et al[23] Diet and Exercise	DasGupta et al[24] Rest	DasGupta et al[24] Exercise	P
Number	25	14	22	21	17		
Gender (F/M)	33/6		12/31		9/8		
Mean age (years)	37 ± 8		46 ± 8	44 ± 7	40 ± 12		
Severity of obesity							
Before	133 ± 8% OW		Weight: 95 ± 10 kg	Weight: 96 ± 11 kg	BMI: 41 ± 8 kg/m²		
After	39 ± 7% OW		Weight: 88 ± 9 kg	Weight: 90 ± 11 kg	BMI: 37 ± 8 kg/m²		
P			<0.001	<0.01			
Mode of weight loss	Gastroplasty		Diet	Diet/Exercise	Diet		
Mode used to assess LV systolic function	Echocardiography		Echocardiography		RNV		
LV fractional shortening (%)							
Before	30 ± 4	24 ± 3	33.4 ± 4.1				
After	33 ± 3	30 ± 4	39.6 ± 5.3				
P	N.S.	<0.01	N.S.				
LVEF (%)							
Before	—	—	—		60 ± 8	+3 ± 5	N.S.
After	—	—	—		58 ± 6	+5 ± 2	<0.0001
P	—	—	—		N.S.	—	

LV = left ventricular; LVFS = left ventricular fractional shortening; LVEF = left ventricular ejection fraction; Vcf = velocity of circumferential fiber shortening; PEP/LVET = pre-ejection period/left ventricular ejection time ratio; OW = overweight; BMI = body mass index; RNV = radionuclide left ventriculography.

Mean values are expressed as ± 1 standard deviation.

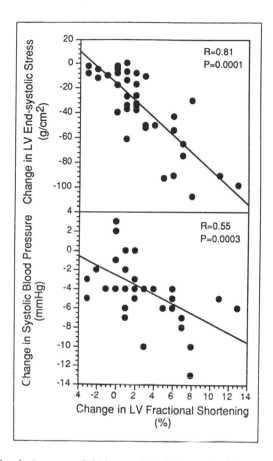

Figure 7. Relation between weight loss-related change in left ventricular fractional shortening (LVFS) and weight loss-related changes in the systolic blood pressure and left ventricular end-systolic wall stress in morbidly obese patients. Weight loss-related change (increase) in LVFS correlated negatively and significantly with weight loss-related changes (decreases) in both of these variables. (Reproduced from *Am J Cardiol* 71:733–737, 1993 with permission.)

verely obese patients and results in improvement in LV exercise reserve in mildly obese patients. Such changes are more likely to occur (but are not limited to) those with impaired LV systolic function prior to weight loss and are attributable, at least in part, to favorable alterations in LV loading conditions (particularly afterload).

In their study of 39 asymptomatic, normotensive, and morbidly obese patients who lost substantial weight following vertical band gastroplasty, Alpert et al.[15] noted that the duration of morbid obesity correlated significantly with the magnitude of weight loss related improvement in LVFS. Duration of morbid obesity also correlated significantly with the magnitude of weight loss-related decrease in the LV internal dimension in diastole, systolic blood pressure, and LV end-systolic wall stress. Thus, it is uncertain whether duration of morbid obesity is an independent predictor of the effect of weight loss on LV systolic function in such individuals. It was noted that most patients whose LVFS improved with weight loss also had LV hypertrophy (increased LV mass/height index).

Summary and Conclusions

LV systolic dysfunction at rest occurs with variable frequency in obese patients. In mildly to moderately obese patients LV systolic function is usually normal. In morbidly obese patients, the incidence of LV systolic dysfunction has been reported to be as high as 36%.[14] Severity of obesity, duration of obesity, and hemodynamic variables that suggest adverse loading conditions predispose to LV systolic dysfunction. LV systolic dysfunction occurs mainly in obese persons with increased LV mass. Whether this is due to myocardial factors, adverse LV loading conditions, or both is uncertain. A relation may exist between LV systolic dysfunction and increased hemostatic function in obese persons.

Exercise produces variable increases in LV systolic dysfunction in most obese individuals. LV exercise reserve is blunted in severely obese persons with increased LV mass and in those who are mildly obese for 120 months or more, but is normal in those with normal LV mass and in those who were mildly obese for less than 120 months. RV exercise reserve is blunted in morbidly obese patients with a high/normal or increased RV internal dimension, but is normal in those with low/mid/normal range RV cavity size.

Weight loss produces an improvement in LV systolic function in morbidly obese patients when it is depressed prior to weight loss, but not in those with normal pre-weight loss LV systolic function. The weight loss-related improvement appears to be related in part to improvement in afterload, even in normotensive patients. Patients with a longer duration of obesity, and those with a higher LV mass, are more likely to experience improvement in LV systolic function than those with a shorter duration of obesity and lower LV mass.

References

1. Wiggers CJ: Studies with consecutive phases of the cardiac cycle I. The duration of the consecutive phases of the cardiac cycle and the criteria for their precise determination. *Am J Physiol* 56:415–438, 1921.
2. Rackley CE: Quantitative evaluation of left ventricular function by radiographic techniques. *Circulation* 54:862–868, 1976.
3. Johns LL, Pohost GM: Nuclear cardiology. In:Schant RC, Alexander RW, O'Rourke RA, et al (eds): *Hurst's The Heart.* 8th ed. McGraw Hill Inc., New York, 1994, pp. 2281–2325.
4. Hagan AD, DeMaria AN: Left ventricular function. In Clinical Applications of Two-Dimensional Echocardiography and Cardiac Doppler, 2nd ed. Little Brown and Company, Boston, 1989, pp 233–260.
5. Scaglione R, Dichiara MA, Indovina R, et al: Left ventricular diastolic and systolic function in normotensive obese subjects: Influence of degree and duration of obesity. *Eur Heart* J 13:138–142, 1992.
6. Merlino G, Scaglione R, Corrao S, et al: Association between reduced lymphocyte β-adrenergic receptors and left ventricular dysfunction in young obese subjects. *Intern J Obes* 18:699–703, 1994.
7. Veille JC, Hanson R: Obesity, pregnancy and left ventricular functioning during the third trimester. *Am J Obstet Gynecol* 171:980–983, 1994.
8. Stoddard MF, Tseuda K, Thomas M, et al: The influence of obesity on left ventricular filling and systolic function. *Am Heart J* 124:694–699, 1992.
9. Messerli FH, Sundgard-Riise K, Reisen ED, et al: Dimorphic cardiac adaptation to obesity and hypertension. *Ann Intern Med* 99:757–761, 1983.
10. Koehler B, Malecka-Tendera E, Drzewiecka B, et al: Evaluation of the cardiovascular system in children with simple obesity. Part II. Echocardiographic assessment. *Mater Med Pol* 2(70):131–133, 1989.
11. Ventura HO, Johnson MR, Grusk B, et al: Cardiac adaptation to obesity and hypertension after heart transplantation. *JACC* 19:55–59, 1992.
12. Alpert MA, Lambert CR, Terry BE, et al: Interrelationship of left ventricular mass, systolic function and diastolic filling in normotensive morbidly obese patients. *Intern J Obes* 19:550–557, 1995.
13. Alexander JK, Woodard CB, Quinones MA, et al: Heart failure from obesity. In Mancini M, Lewis B, Contaldo F (eds): *Medical Complications of Obesity.* Academic Press, London, 1978, pp. 179–187.
14. Alpert MA, Terry BE, Lambert CR, et al: Factors influencing left ventricular systolic function in non-hypertensive morbidly obese patients, and effect of weight loss induced by gastroplasty. *Am J Cardiol* 71:733–737, 1993.
15. Alpert MA, Lambert CR, Panayiotou H, et al: Relation of duration of morbid obesity to left ventricular mass, systolic function and diastolic filling and effect of weight loss. *Am J Cardiol* 76:1194–1197, 1995.
16. Nakajima T, Fujoka S, Tokunaga K, et al: Non-invasive study of left ventricular performance in obese patients: Influence of duration of obesity. *Circulation* 71:4481–486, 1985.
17. Alpert MA, Terry BE, Mulekar M, et al: Cardiac morphology and left ventricular function in normotensive morbidly obese patents with and with-

out congestive heart failure and effect of weight loss. *Am J Cardiol,* in press.

18. Licata G, Scaglione R, Avellone G, et al: Hemostatic function in young subjects with central obesity: Relationship with left ventricular function. *Metabolism* 44:1417–1421, 1995.

19. Licata G, Scaglione R, Paterna S, et al: Left ventricular function response to exercise in normotensive obese subjects: Influence of degree and duration of obesity. *J Obesity* 37:223–230, 1992.

20. Alaud-din A, Meterissian S, Lisbona R, et al: Assessment of cardiac function in patients who were morbidly obese. *Surgery* 108:809–820, 1990.

21. Alpert MA, Singh A, Terry BE, et al: Effect of exercise on left ventricular systolic function and reserve in morbid obesity. *Am J Cardiol* 63:1478–1482, 1989.

22. Alpert MA, Singh A, Terry BE, et al: Effect of exercise and cavity size on right ventricular function in morbid obesity. *Am J Cardiol* 64:1361–1365, 1989.

23. Wirth A, Kröger H: Improvement of left ventricular morphology and function in obese subjects following a diet and exercise program. *Intern J Obes* 19:61–66, 1995.

24. Das Gupta P, Ramhanmdany E, Bridgen G, et al: Improvement of left ventricular function after rapid weight loss in obesity. *Eur Heart J* 13:1060–1066, 1992.

Chapter 7

Obesity, Hypertension, and the Heart

Efrain Reisin, MD
and M. Eileen Cook, MD

Introduction

Obesity refers to a surplus in body fat[1] and is defined by some authors as any weight that is 20% above ideal body weight, or as a body mass index that is higher than 27.8 for men and 27.3 for women.[2] Obesity now affects one-third of all Americans, which is up from just over one-fourth during the last decade.[2] Since hypertension and obesity are directly related,[3, 4] and since the direct correlation between the height of arterial pressure and the magnitude of body weight cannot be explained as an artifact of false blood pressure readings induced by arm girth,[5] this increase in the incidence of obesity has significant public health implications.

Underlying mechanisms that account for the increased presence of elevated blood pressure in the obese population are the subject of extensive discussion in medical literature. Obesity alone has been linked to expanded blood volume and increased cardiac output. Hypertension develops if systemic vascular resistance fails to decrease as cardiac output increases.[6] Other abnormalities linked to obesity include dysregulation of metabolic and neuroendocrine systems (Figure 1).[6, 7]

From: Alpert MA, and Alexander JK, (eds). *The Heart and Lung in Obesity*. Armonk, NY: Futura Publishing Company, Inc., © 1998.

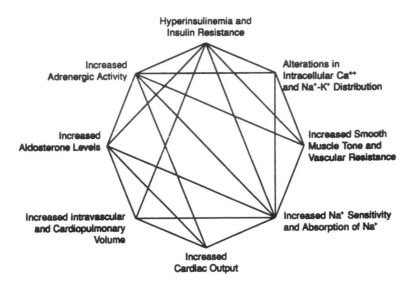

Figure 1. Physiological mechanisms involved in obesity-hypertension. (Modified from Reference 6 with permission.)

Epidemiology and Heredity

Several cross-sectional[3,8,9] and longitudinal[4,10,11] epidemiological studies have demonstrated a direct relation between obesity and hypertension. Chiang et al.[12] reviewed 31 reports from 15 nations representing all continents; they demonstrated that in different populations, weight gain and increase in blood pressure occurred with age. The association between blood pressure and weight tends to be higher in populations where obesity is common. These investigators proposed that weight gain acted as an environmental stress that caused hypertension in genetically predisposed individuals. Their findings were confirmed by a study that revealed that populations with the lowest age-related rise in blood pressure were those with lower average weights.[13]

However, the prevalence of hypertension in obese patients varies in different studies. For example, among the most obese patients in the Framingham Study, 46% were hypertensive.[3] Van Itallie[14] reviewed data from the Second National Health and Nutrition Examination Survey to determine the relative risk of hypertension due to excess weight. Among all survey respondents, the risk for hypertension was three times greater in the obese. Obese young adults had a relative risk of hypertension 5.6 times higher than that of the nonobese young adults. The relative risk fell to 1.9 times in respondents 45 to 75 years of age. Van Itallie[14] also noted that although African-American women tend to be more obese than white women, obesity increased the risk of hypertension only 1.5 times among African-American women, compared with 2.6 times in white women. Johnson et al.[15] noted that a follow-up survey of patients age 15 to 29 years of age, conducted several years after the initial investigation, revealed that hypertension was more common in the second examination and correlated with body mass index in white males, white females, and African-American females, but not in African-American males.

The difference in the risk of hypertension found in diverse obese populations may be explained by studies that have shown a higher incidence of hypertension in individuals with upper body obesity than in those with lower body obesity.[3,8,9] Upper body obesity also may be important in any consideration of risk factors for mortality. A large epidemiological study[16] showed that central adiposity, rather than body mass index, is a key risk factor for death due to coronary artery disease in women. Mortality also was related to other predictors such as hypertension, diabetes mellitus, cigarette smoking, and the postmenopausal state.[16] Two European surveys arrived at a similar conclusion, which indicates that high levels of obesity were only marginally associated with excess mortality alone, but became a health risk when associated with elevated serum triglycerides, hypertension, and abdominal adiposity.[17,18]

Several genes that contribute to cardiovascular regulation or body mass index may be involved in the development and maintenance of obesity-related hypertension.[19] Selby et al.[20] examined the association of the low-density lipoprotein (LDL), subclass phenotype with plasma insulin levels, and with other aspects of the insulin-resistance syndrome (a mechanism linked to obesity-hypertension) in a group of 206 monozygous and 196 dizygous twin pairs of women. The authors concluded that LDL is an integral feature of the insulin-resistance syndrome and that nongenetic factors, either behavioral or environmental, are important for the expression of the phenotype.[20]

However, Herzog et al.[19] examined the neuropeptide-Y Y1-receptor gene (NPY Y1R) for involvement in hypertension and obesity. Although NPY Y1R increases blood pressure and appetite, the authors did not find an association between the NPY Y1R receptor gene, essential hypertension, and obesity.[19]

Mechanisms in Obesity-hypertension, Insulin Resistance, and Hyperinsulinemia

One explanation for the increased incidence of hypertension in obesity is the widely held belief that hyperinsulinemia accompanies obesity. Several epidemiological studies demonstrated that hypertension is prevalent in 30% to 50% of diabetics, which is approximately double the incidence of hypertension in the general population.[21–23]

The insulin-obesity-hypertension relation appears to be more evident in subjects with upper body obesity. In these individuals, hyperinsulemia is the result of a large accumulation of lipolytic hyperactive abdominal cells, with a release of a large amount of free fatty acids into the portal vein. These changes trigger excessive hepatic synthesis of triglyceride, inhibition of insulin uptake, hyperinsulinemia, and insulin resistance.[24,25] Istfan et al.[26] measured the degree of association among obesity, blood pressure, insulin resistance, and insulin secretion in 72 obese-hypertensive, obese-nonhypertensive, and normal-weight-normotensive control subjects. Insulin's action on glucose uptake was inversely associated with blood pressure status, weight, and age. Multivariate regression analysis indicated that the percentage of body fat and the waist/hip ratio had the strongest correlation with insulin action on glucose uptake. Obese-hypertensives had a significantly lower index of insulin action compared with the obese-nonhypertensives or the normal weight subjects. However, this association remains controversial, since other epidemiological studies failed to show a consistent relation between hypertension and hyperinsulinemia.[27] Others argue that the effect of insulin on blood pressure may be short term and cannot explain sustained hypertension,[28] or that genetic and environmental factors explain the conflicting data.[29,30] Hall and colleagues[31] note the lack of studies on long-term renal and cardiovascular responses to insulin infusion in man. The few long-term studies conducted in animals, and the chronic hyperinsulinemia associated with insulinomas, do not support the idea that hyperinsulinemia is the major cause of hypertension.[31]

Research studies in rats have shown that administration of insulin increases the vascular wall thickness of myocardial arterioles by causing hypertrophy of the tunica media,[32] which may lead to changes in the cardiovascular system and result in hypertension. Insulin infused into the renal artery increases sodium reabsorption in the diluting segment of the distal nephron, which leads to sodium retention.[33] Accordingly, resistance to insulin can result in sodium retention, hypervolemia, and increased peripheral vascular resistance.[32–34]

The Renin-Angiotensin-Aldosterone System

Plasma renin activity has been shown to be unchanged or reduced in inverse proportion to weight.[35,36] Hiramatasu et al.[35] has suggested that aldosterone may play a role in obesity-hypertension. These investigators measured plasma renin activity and aldosterone concentrations in 85 patients whose weight varied from less than 10% to more than 49% of their ideal weight. The ratio of plasma aldosterone to plasma renin activity increased with weight gain because plasma renin activity fell progressively. The net effect of this was an increase in total body sodium and water.[7,36] However, Rocchini and colleagues[37] studied salt-sensitive blood pressure changes in obese and nonobese adolescents and found higher plasma aldosterone concentrations in the obese subjects, although plasma renin values were similar in both groups.

Sodium, Sympathetic Activity, and NA⁺-K⁺ ATPase Activity

Previous studies have shown that increased sodium intake is a major factor in hypertension in the obese patient,[38] and obesity appears to promote salt sensitivity.[39] The exact pathogenic mechanism that links sodium intake and salt sensitivity to obesity-hypertension remains unknown, although insulin resistance appears to be a common metabolic link.[30,40]

Salt sensitivity predisposes the individual to renal failure.[40] Campese[40] proposed that renal alterations are induced by a decrease in renal blood flow and an increase in filtration fraction and intraglomerular pressure. These changes will induce glomerulosclerosis.[40] However, in the obese population, more studies are necessary to verify that these alterations occur (Figure 2).

Cortisol production and urinary excretion of cortisol increase in obesity, but are proportional to the increase in body size. However, plasma concentrations of cortisol are generally within normal ranges.[35]

A recent investigation[41] performed in a cross-sectional study of nondiabetic men showed a 10% increase in hypertension among participants in the lowest tertiles of both insulin and norepinephrine levels, compared with a 35% increase among participants in the highest tertiles of these variables. These findings suggest that insulin levels and sympathetic nervous system activity are associated with hypertension among middle-age and elderly men.[41]

Obese-hypertensives have decreased activity of Na-K-ATPase in their erythrocytes, which results in lower levels of intracellular sodium,

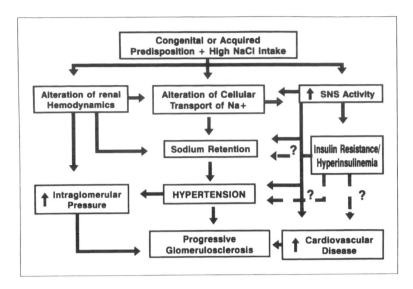

Figure 2. Salt sensitivity and cardiovascular and renal complications. (Reproduced from Reference 40 with permission.)

and may cause decreased calcium efflux, which results in higher intracellular calcium concentration.[42–44] When these changes occur in smooth muscle cells, they may increase vascular tone and peripheral resistance.[37,45,46]

Plasma, Total Blood Volume, and Systemic Hemodynamics

Increased plasma volume has been implicated as an important mechanism that triggers other hemodynamic changes and induces obesity-hypertension.[6,36,47–49] In patients with essential hypertension, renovascular hypertension, or pheochromocytoma, plasma and total blood volumes progressively contract as arterial pressure and total peripheral resistance increase.[49] In contrast, other forms of hypertension are directly related to the height of arterial pressure and the magnitude of intravascular volume, specifically in patients with renal parenchymal disease, low renin hypertension, and steroid-dependent forms of hypertension.[49]

Several studies demonstrated that, in obese-hypertensive patients, plasma and total blood volumes increased when absolute values were considered.[36,47,48] However, the distribution of intravascular volume is dependent on the distribution of body fat.[49] Adipose tissue is apparently underperfused compared with lean tissue,[36] and the ratio of intravascular volume to body weight decreases as total body fat increases.[36,50] This absolute increase in intravascular volume in obese-hypertensives represents the actual volume pumped by the heart and redistributed centrally to the cardiopulmonary area and thereby increasing venous return and cardiac output.[51]

One previous study,[52] which showed the indices of the partition of plasma fluid volume/interstitial fluid volume and intracellular fluid volume/interstitial fluid volume, reported that the plasma fluid volume/interstitial fluid volume ratio was normal in obese-hypertensive patients and correlated negatively with mean arterial pressure. These investigators also demonstrated that intracellular body water/interstitial fluid volume was increased in obese-hypertensive subjects. They concluded that this might be caused either by an intracellular body water level too high for the level of interstitial fluid volume, or by an interstitial fluid level too low for the level of intracellular body water.

Earlier studies of obese-hypertensives have shown increased cardiac output and stroke volume.[47,48,53] These results were confirmed in a group of obese-hypertensives compared with normotensive obese subjects.[36] Some authors have reported low total resistance,[54] which suggests that patients with obesity-related hypertension are hemodynamically younger in terms of systemic circulation, when compared with lean hypertensive subjects. Other studies describe a second type of obese-hypertensive patients in whom hypertension and obesity are more likely associated, but not closely related. These patients are characterized by elevated peripheral resistance.[55] We believe that hypertension develops in obese hypertensives if systemic vascular resistance fails to decrease as cardiac output increases,[49] and we agree with studies that have shown that peripheral resistance was inappropriately normal in obese-hypertensive patients, when compared with that in normotensive subjects.[36]

The Effect of Obesity-Hypertension on the Heart

In obese subjects, the high circulating volume and stroke volume enhance left ventricular (LV) volume and LV filling pressure.[6] The increase in preload to the left atrium and LV induces atrial and ventricular dilation, which are findings described by echocardiographic studies. In accordance with La Place's law, however, LV dilation also increases wall stress and, therefore, afterload.[56] In obesity, the LV adapts by increasing muscle mass and thickening the myocardial wall.[57] These echocardiographic findings were corroborated by earlier studies of obese subjects on autopsy that showed increased cardiac weight associated with thickened, hypertrophied ventricles.[58]

Echocardiographic changes in other chambers in obese-normotensive and obese-hypertensive subjects showed increased diastolic, systolic, and aortic root diameters.[59] These augmented diameters are related to the volume overload imposed by the hemodynamic characteristics previously described in obesity-hypertension.[36]

In obese individuals, the myocardium adapts to chamber dilation by adding contractile elements in series. The myocardium also must thicken to restore wall stress to normal, a process that also adds contractile elements in parallel[59,60]; this adaptive process results in eccentric LV hypertrophy, a characteristic finding in obese-normotensive subjects.[56,61–64]

The prevalence of LV hypertrophy increases with age and is ten times higher in patients with hypertension than in normotensive subjects.[65] The pathogenesis of these changes is still controversial, but may be influenced by demographic (e.g., sex, age, and race), exogenous (e.g., salt and alcohol intake), and neurohumoral (e.g., insulin, growth hormone, angiotensin, and sympathetic activity) factors[64,65] (Figure 3). In

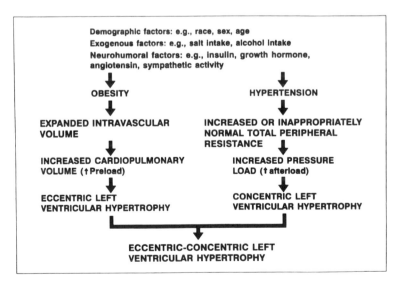

Figure 3. The effect of obesity-hypertension on the heart. (Modified from Reference 49 with permission.)

these patients, the increase in ventricular wall stress without cardiac dilatation induces at the myocardial level an addition of contractile elements in parallel only.[64] A response to an increased afterload will cause concentric LV hypertrophy.

The coexistence of obesity and hypertension will increase the pre-load and enhance end-diastolic volume and LV filling pressure. These changes take place in a ventricle already altered by an increased after-load due to arterial hypertension and will cause eccentric-concentric LV hypertrophy,[56] a phenomenon that increases the risk of congestive heart failure (CHF)[51] (Figures 3 and 4).

The presence of LV hypertrophy is also a risk factor for the devel-opment of cardiac arrhythmias (e.g., atrial fibrillation).[65,66] Recent in-vestigations on obese subjects have reported the presence of mononu-clear cell infiltration in and around the sinoatrial node and/or its approaches, with marked fat throughout the conduction system.[67] These changes may explain the high rates of sudden unexpected car-diac death in patients with morbid obesity.[68]

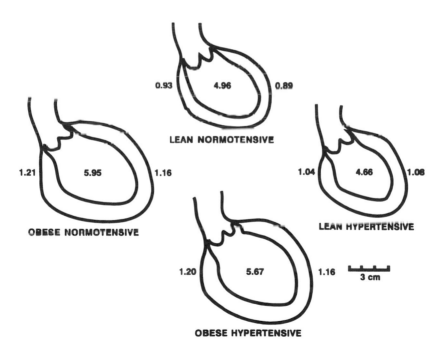

Figure 4. Left ventricular dimensions in lean and obese subjects. (Reproduced from Reference 56 with permission.)

Hypertension and obesity also generate other clinical implications. LV hypertrophy alters coronary circulation, which decreases myocardial vasculature during periods of increased blood flow demand and increases the incidence of coronary heart disease.[65]

Other authors[40] considered that the salt sensitivity present in obese subjects may interrelate alterations of cellular transport of sodium with some of the hemodynamic and hormonal abnormalities previously described in obese subjects.[39] These mechanisms trigger greater cardiovascular morbidity and mortality.[40]

In summary, several epidemiological studies have shown a direct relation between obesity and hypertension and, specifically, between upper body obesity and hypertension. These investigations have also demonstrated that central adiposity is an important risk factor for death from coronary heart disease.

A series of endocrine, adrenergic, and metabolic mechanisms have been linked to the development of obesity-hypertension. These include: insulin resistance; hyperinsulinemia; increases in adrenergic activity; and increases in aldosterone levels, which induce sodium and water retention and, consequently, hypervolemia. These changes affect some hemodynamic characteristics of the obese-hypertensive patient such as: absolute total blood volume, with higher redistribution to the cardiopulmonary volume, which enhances venous return; cardiac output stroke volume; and LV wall thickness, with peripheral resistance that is inappropriately normal in the context of increased cardiac output.

These hemodynamic alterations enhance the preload to the LV, which induces eccentric LV hypertrophy. Hypertension will increase the afterload, which induces concentric LV hypertrophy. The coexistence of obesity and hypertension will induce eccentric-concentric LV hypertrophy, which enhances the risk of CHF.

Acknowledgments

The authors thank Steve Gavigan, R.N. for his valuable help and Anne Compliment for her excellent editorial assistance.

References

1. Bray GA: *Obesity in America.* NIH, Washington, DC, 1980, pp. 1–19.
2. Kuczmarski RJ, Flegal KM, Campbell SM, et al: Increasing prevalence of

overweight among US adults. The National Health and Nutrition Examination Surveys, 1960–1991. *JAMA* 272:205–211, 1994.

3. Kannel WB, Brand N, Skinner JJ, et al: The relation of adiposity to blood pressure and development of hypertension: The Framingham study. *Ann Intern Med* 67:48–49, 1967.

4. Hsu PH, Mathewson FAL, Rabkin SW: Blood pressure and body mass index pattern: A longitudinal study. *J Chronic Disease* 30:93–113, 1977.

5. Forsberg SA, Guzman MD, Berlund S: Validity of blood pressure measurement with cuff in the arm and forearm. *Acta Med Scand* 188:389–396, 1970.

6. Reisin E: Obesity hypertension: Non pharmacologic and pharmacologic therapeutic modalities. In Laragh JH, Brenner BM (eds): *Hypertension: Pathophysiology, Diagnosis and Management,* 2nd ed. Raven Press, New York, 1995, pp. 2683–2691.

7. Dustan HP: Obesity and hypertension. *Diabetes Care* 14:488–504, 1991.

8. Stamler R, Stamler J, Riedlinger WF, et al: Weight and blood pressure findings in hypertension screening of 1 million Americans. *JAMA* 240:1607–1620, 1978.

9. Epstein FH: Prevalence of chronic disease and distribution of selected physiological variables in a total community of Tecumseh, Michigan. *Am J Epidemiol* 81:307–322, 1965.

10. Levi RL, White PD, Stroud WD: Overweight: A prognostic significance in relation to hypertension and cardiovascular renal diseases. *JAMA* 121:951–953, 1946.

11. Rabkin SW, Mathewson FAL, Hsu PH: Relation of body weight to development of ischemic heart disease in a cohort of young North American men after a 26-year observation period. The Manitoba Study. *Am J Cardiol* 399:452–458, 1977.

12. Chiang BN, Perlman LV, Epstein FM: Overweight and hypertension. Circulation 39:403–410, 1969.

13. Epstein FM, Eckhoff RD: Epidemiology of high blood pressure, geographic distributions and etiologic factors. In Stamler J, Stamler R, Pullman TN (eds): *Epidemiology of Hypertension.* Grune and Stratten, New York, 1967, pp. 155–166.

14. Van Itallic TB: The problem of obesity: Health implications of overweight and obesity in the United States. *Ann Intern Med* 103:983–988, 1985.

15. Johnson AL, Cornoni JC, Cassel JC, et al: Influence of race, sex, and weight on blood pressure behavior in young adults. *Am J Cardiol* 35:523–530, 1975.

16. Prineas RJ, Folsom AR, Kaye SA: Central obesity and increased risk of coronary artery disease mortality in older women. *Ann Epidemiol* 3:35–41, 1993.

17. Bengtsson C, Bjorkelund C, Lapidus L, et al: Associations of serum lipid concentrations and obesity with mortality in women: 20 year follow-up of participants in prospective population study in Gothenburg, Sweden. *Br Med J* 307:1385–1388, 1993.

18. Menotti A, Descovich GC, Lauti M, et al: Indexes of obesity and all-causes mortality in Italian epidemiological data. *Prev Med* 22:L293-L303, 1993.

19. Herzog H, Selbie LA, Zee RYL, et al: Neuropeptide-Y Y1 receptor gene polymorphism: Cross-sectional analysis in essential hypertension and obesity. *Biochem Biophys Res Comm* 196:902–906, 1993.

20. Selby JV, Austin MA, Newman B, et al: LDL subclass phenotypes and the insulin resistance syndrome in women. *Circulation* 88:381–387, 1993.
21. Christlieb AR: Diabetes and hypertensive vascular disease. Mechanisms and treatment. *Am J Cardiol* 32:592–606, 1973.
22. Kannel WB, McGee DL: Diabetes and cardiovascular risk factors: The Framingham Study. *Circulation* 59:8–13, 1979.
23. Zemel MB: Insulin resistance, obesity and hypertension: An overview. *J Nutr* 125:S171–S175, 1975.
24. Janet RJ, Keen H, McCartney M, et al: Glucose tolerance and blood pressure in two population samples: Their relationship to diabetes mellitus and hypertension. *J Epidemiol* 7:15–24, 1978.
25. Krotkiewski M, Bjorntorp P, Sjostrom L, et al: Impact of obesity on metabolism in men and women: Importance of regional adipose tissue distribution. *J Clin Invest* 72:1150–1162, 1983.
26. Istfan NW, Plaisted CS, Bistrian BR, et al: Insulin resistance versus insulin secretion in the hypertension of obesity. *Hypertension* 19:385–392, 1992.
27. Maxwell MH, Heber D, Waks AV, et al: Role of insulin and norepinephrine in the hypertension of obesity. *Am J Hypertens* 7:402–408, 1995.
28. Hall JE, Brands MW, Zappe DH, et al: Insulin resistance, hyperinsulinemia, and hypertension: Causes, consequences, or merely correlations? *Proc Soc Exp Biol Med* 208:317–329, 1995.
29. Landsberg L: Insulin and hypertension. *Proc Soc Exp Biol Med* 208:315–316, 1995.
30. Mark AL, Anderson EA: Genetic factors determine the blood pressure response to insulin resistance and hyperinsulinemia: A call to refocus the insulin hypothesis of hypertension. *Proc Soc Exp Biol Med* 208:330–336, 1995.
31. Hall JE, Summers RL, Brands MW, et al: Resistance to the metabolic action of insulin and its role in hypertension. *Am J Hypertens* 7:772–788, 1994.
32. Zimlichman R, Zeidel L, Gefel D, et al: Insulin induces medial hypertrophy of myocardial arterioles in rats. *Am J Hypertens* 8:915–920, 1995.
33. DeFronzo RA, Cooke RA, Andres R, et al: The effect of insulin on renal handling of sodium, potassium, calcium, and phosphate in man. *J Clin Invest* 55:845–855, 1975.
34. Feldman RD, Hramiak IM, Finegood DT, et al: Parallel regulation of the local vascular and systemic metabolic effects of insulin. *J Clin Endocrinol Metab* 80:1556–1559, 1995.
35. Hiramatzu K, Yamada T, Ichikawa K, et al: Changes in endocrine activities relative to obesity in patients with essential hypertension. *J Am Geriatr Soc* 29:25–30, 1981.
36. Messerli FH, Christie B, DeCarvalho GR, et al: Obesity and essential hypertension, intravascular volume, sodium excretion and plasma renin activity. *Arch Intern Med* 141:81–85, 1981.
37. Rocchini AP, Key J, Bondie D, et al: The effect of weight loss on the sensitivity of blood pressure to sodium on obese adolescents. *N Engl J Med* 321:580–585, 1989.
38. Dahl KK, Silver L, Christie RW: Role of salt in the fall of blood pressure accompanying reduction of obesity. *N Engl J Med* 258:1186–1192, 1958.

39. Rocchini AP: The relationship of sodium sensitivity to insulin resistance. *Am J Med* Sci 307:575–580, 1994.
40. Campese V: Salt sensitivity in hypertension. Renal and cardiovascular implications. *Hypertension* 23:531–550, 1994.
41. Ward CD, Spanow D, Landsberg L, et al: Influence of insulin, sympathetic nervous system and obesity on blood pressure: The normotensive aging study. *J Hypertens* 14:301–308, 1996.
42. De Luise M, Blackburn CL, Flier JS: Reduced activity of the red-cell sodium-potassium pump in human obesity. *N Engl J Med* 303:1017–1022, 1980.
43. Klimes I, Nagulesparan M, Unger RH, et al: Decreased Na$^+$ K$^+$ ATPase activity in erythrocyte membranes and intact erythrocytes from obese men. *J Clin Endocrinol Metab* 54:721–724, 1982.
44. Avenell A, Leeds AR: Sodium intake inhibition of Na+ K+ ATPase and obesity. *Lancet* 1:836, 1981.
45. Boehringer K, Beretta-Piccoli C, Weidmann P, et al: Pressor factors and cardiovascular pressor responsiveness in lean and overweight normal or hypertensive subjects. *Hypertension* 4:697–702, 1982.
46. Sowers JR, Niby M, Stern N, et al: Blood pressure and hormone changes associated with weight reduction in the obese. *Hypertension* 4:686–691, 1982.
47. Alexander JK: Obesity and the circulation. *Mod Cardiovasc Dis* 32: 799–803, 1963.
48. Alexander JK, Dennis EW, Smith WG, et al: Blood volume, cardiac output, and distribution of systemic blood flow in extreme obesity. *Cardiovas Res Center Bull* 1:39–44, 1962.
49. Reisin E, Frohlich ED: Hemodynamics in obesity. In Zanchetti A, Tarazi RC (eds): *Handbook of Hypertension, Vol 7. Pathophysiology of Hypertension—Cardiovascular Aspects.* Elsevier Science Publishers, Amsterdam, The Netherlands, 1986, pp. 280–297.
50. Feldschuch J, Enson Y: Prediction of the normal blood volume: Relation of blood volume to body habitus. *Circulation* 56:605–612, 1977.
51. Frohlich ED, Messerli FH, Reisin E, et al: The problem of obesity and hypertension. Response to hypertension therapy. *Hypertension* 5(Suppl III): III71–III78, 1983.
52. Raison J, Achimastos J, London G, et al: Intravascular volume, extracellular fluid volume and total body water in obese and non obese hypertensive patients. *Am J Cardiol* 51:165–170, 1983.
53. Backman L, Freyschuss V, Hallberg D, et al: Cardiovascular function in extreme obesity. *Acta Med Scand* 193:437–446, 1973.
54. Schmieder RE, Messerli FH: Does obesity influence early target organ damage in hypertensive patients? *Circulation* 87:1482–1488, 1993.
55. Ferrannini E: The hemodynamic of obesity: A theoretical analysis. *J Hypertens* 10:1411–1423, 1992.
56. Messerli FH, Sundgaard-Riise K, Reisin E, et al: Dimorphic cardiac adaptation to obesity and arterial hypertension. *Ann Intern Med* 99:757–761, 1983.
57. Chakko S, Mayor M, Allison MD, et al: Abnormal left ventricular diastolic filling in eccentric left ventricular hypertrophy of obesity. *Am J Cardiol* 68:95–98, 1991.

58. Amad KH, Brennan JC, Alexander JK: The cardiac pathology of chronic exogenous obesity. *Circulation* 32:740–745, 1965.
59. Messerli FH, Sundgaard-Riise K, Reisin E, et al: Disparate cardiovascular effects of obesity and arterial hypertension. *Am J Med* 74:808–812, 1983.
60. Lauer MS, Anderson KM, Kannel WB, et al: The impact of obesity on left ventricular mass and geometry. The Framingham Heart Study. *JAMA* 266:231–236, 1991.
61. Reisin E, Messerli FH: Obesity-related hypertension: Mechanisms, cardiovascular risks, and heredity. *Curr Opin Nephrol-Hyperten* 4: 67–71, 1995.
62. Dustan HP: Hypertension and obesity. *Prim Care* 18:495–507, 1991.
63. Reisin E, Frohlich ED: Cardiovascular changes in obese hypertensive patients. *Prim Cardiol* 12:79–84, 1986.
64. Frohlich ED, Epstein C, Chobanian AV, et al: The heart in hypertension. *N Engl J Med* 327:998–1008, 1992.
65. Lip GYH, Gammage MD, Beevers DG: Hypertension and the heart. *BM Bull* 50:299–321, 1994.
66. De la Maza MP, Estevez A, Bunout D, et al: Ventricular mass in hypertensive obese subjects. *Int J Obes Relat Disord* 18:193–197, 1994.
67. Bharati S, Lev M: Cardiac conduction system involvement in sudden death of obese young people. *Am Heart J* 129:273–281, 1995.
68. Duflou J, Virmani R, Robin J, et al: Sudden death as a result of heart disease in morbid obesity. *Am Heart J* 130:306–313, 1995.

Chapter 8

Obesity and Pulmonary Function

Dudley F. Rochester, MD

Introduction

Morbid obesity has a significant impact on the respiratory system, with alterations in pulmonary gas exchange, respiratory mechanics, pulmonary function, exercise capacity, respiratory muscle strength, and the control of breathing. A subgroup of these patients may develop the obesity hypoventilation syndrome (OHS) with hypercapnia. Both groups often complain of exercise intolerance and dyspnea on exertion, and both are prone to develop obstructive sleep apnea (OSA). In addition, both groups are at increased risk for developing postoperative complications such as pneumonia, hypoxemia, and atelectasis. This chapter summarizes the alterations in respiratory and ventilatory physiology consequent to simple obesity, and indicates the differences between simple obesity and OHS. Aspects of relations between obesity, OHS, and OSA will be reviewed, and approaches to treatment of morbid obesity and OHS will be outlined.

Body Composition

An appreciation of the methods used to qualify obesity,[1-5] assess the amount and distribution of body fat,[6-19] and estimate fat free mass[6, 11, 20-22] is essential in understanding the impact of obesity on pulmonary function. A detailed discussion of these methods is contained in the Appendix of this book.

From: Alpert MA, and Alexander JK, (eds). *The Heart and Lung in Obesity*. Armonk, NY: Futura Publishing Company, Inc., © 1998.

Gas Exchange and Pulmonary Function

Gas Exchange

Severely obese patients are often hypoxemic with a widened alveolar-arterial oxygen tension gradient (A-aPO$_2$),[23–31] but hypoxemia may be mild or absent.[23,27,32–36] The PaO$_2$ is most apt to be abnormal when obese subjects are supine, even if it is normal when they are sitting or standing.[27, 37] Hypoxemia in obesity results from a mismatch of ventilation and perfusion. The lung bases are well perfused, but they are underventilated due to airway closure and alveolar collapse.[33, 38–40] This effect is most pronounced in obese subjects with small lung volumes[41] and in the supine position.[42]

The single breath diffusing capacity (DLCO) is normal in simple obesity[3, 29, 33, 43–46] and slightly reduced in OHS.[33, 43, 47] The physiological dead space (VD), the ratio of VD to tidal volume (VD/VT) and pulmonary mixing as judged from nitrogen washout are normal.[32,34,43,48]

Typical values for blood gas composition are summarized in Table 1. The majority of patients with severe obesity are eucapnic, even though obesity produces a greater demand upon the ventilatory system to maintain a normal PaCO$_2$. Patients with OHS are hypercapnic and have a lower PaO$_2$ than patients with simple obesity.[28, 30–33, 49] The A-aPO$_2$ is somewhat larger in OHS, but most of the reduction of PaO$_2$ re-

---

Table 1
Gas Exchange in Normals (NL), Obese Subjects (OB),
and Obesity Hypoventilation Syndrome (OHS)

Variable	Units	NL	OB	OHS
PaCO$_2$	(torr)	38	39	51
PaO$_2$	(torr)	89	80	59
AaPO$_2$	(torr)	15	23	27
DL$_{CO}$	(mL/min/torr)	35	30	25

PaCO$_2$ = pressure of carbon dioxide in arterial blood; PaO$_2$ = pressure of oxygen in arterial blood; AaPO$_2$ = oxygen pressure difference between alveolar gas and arterial blood; DL$_{CO}$ = diffusing capacity for carbon monoxide.

sults from the increase in $PaCO_2$. The $PaCO_2$ falls with hyperventilation, but the extent to which it falls is related to the FEV_1 (% predicted)[50], therefore, the mechanical impediments to breathing also contribute to hypercapnia in OHS.

Spirometry and Lung Volumes

Simple obesity, uncomplicated by upper or lower airway obstruction, generally exerts only mild effects on pulmonary function. The most frequent abnormality is reduction of the expiratory reserve volume (ERV), because the obese abdomen displaces the diaphragm into the chest. In normal weight and mildly obese males ERV was inversely proportional to body mass index (BMI), even though all other lung volumes were normal.[51] Ray et al.[3] studied 43 healthy, young, and nonsmoking obese subjects whose body weight (BW) averaged 159 kg. Their weight/height (HT) ratio was 0.93 kg/cm, which corresponds to a BMI of 54 kg/m^2. The ERV was approximately 60% of normal when BW/HT exceeded 0.7 kg/cm and 35% normal when BW/HT exceeded 1 kg/cm. The vital capacity (VC), functional residual capacity (FRC), total lung capacity (TLC), and maximal voluntary ventilation (MVV) were within the normal range in most of these subjects. In the severely obese with BW/HT was greater than 1 kg/cm (BMI > 60 kg/m^2), the VC was reduced by 25%, and MVV was reduced by 31%, but there was no reduction in FRC or TLC.[3] Mildly obese men whose obesity is more centrally distributed have lower values of FVC, FEV_1, and TLC than those with more peripheral obesity.[14] Thus, the adverse effects of obesity on pulmonary function cannot be entirely explained by the absolute load of adipose tissue on the chest wall as similar degrees of obesity in simple obesity and OHS result in different patterns of lung volume changes.

Summary of Pulmonary Function Tests

Results of multiple studies are summarized in Figure 1.[3,10,23,26,28,30,31,33,36,43,52] The deficits tend to be more severe in OHS (where TLC is approximately 20% smaller) and VC, FEV_1, and MVV are approximately 40% smaller than in simple obesity. The ERV in OHS is equivalent to the most severe cases of simple obesity. The FRC is 75% to 80% predicted in OHS.

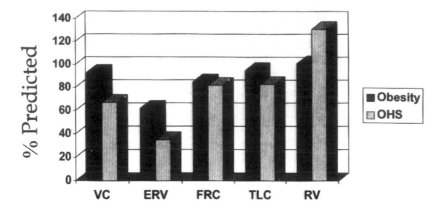

Figure 1. Typical values for lung volumes (% predicted) in patients with simple obesity and obesity hypoventilation syndrome. See text for sources.

Respiratory System Mechanics

Compliance

Some investigators have found that chest wall or total respiratory system compliance is reduced in obesity,[35,47,53] but others have found little deviation from normal in simple obesity. Values for compliance of the chest wall vary as a function of technique and the degree of respiratory muscle relaxation. Sharp et al.[43] found that compliance of the chest wall and total respiratory system in simple obesity were 92% and 80%, respectively, of values obtained in normal subjects. By way of contrast, compliance of the chest wall and total respiratory system were 37% and 44% of normal, respectively, in patients with OHS[43] (i.e., substantially lower than in simple obesity). Part of the decrement in respiratory system compliance results from a fall in lung compliance, which is decreased by approximately 25% in simple obesity and 40% in OHS.[43, 54] Some of the reduction may be due to the increased pulmonary blood volume[24] and some to increased closure of dependent airways.[25]

It is commonly believed that the chest wall is stiff and noncompliant because of the increased weight pressing upon the thorax and abdomen. The excess weight does present an added inspiratory load, but it is of the threshold type, that is, a weight that has to be lifted to inspire. This can be demonstrated by measuring chest wall or respiratory system compliance with the pulse airflow technique. The threshold load appears as if it were a resistance to flow, and the chest wall compliance per se is relatively normal in simple obesity, even when BW/HT and BMI are as high as 1.2 kg/cm and 80 kg/m, respectively.[55]

Resistance

Airway, chest wall, and respiratory system resistances are elevated in simple obesity and are higher in patients with a higher BMI.[43,56] The major reason for increased lung and respiratory system resistance in obesity is the reduction of lung volume. There is a high degree of correlation between airway conductance and FRC and, after correcting for the reduced lung volume, specific airway conductance may be near normal or reduced to 50% to 70% of normal.[56, 57] Chest wall and total respiratory system resistances are also increased in simple obesity and OHS, with the chest wall and respiratory systems resistances being higher in OHS.[43] Sharp et al.[43] found that lung resistance in OHS is the same as in simple obesity, but chest wall and total respiratory resistances are higher. Total respiratory system resistance measured using the forced oscillation technique is higher and reactance is lower in simple obesity as compared to normal.[58] Respiratory resistance rises and reactance falls when obese subjects shift from upright to supine.[58]

In the absence of underlying lung disease, the ratio FEV_1/FVC is normal in patients with simple obesity and OHS,[3,10,23,29-31, 33,35,36,43,49,52,56] even when their lung resistance is high.[43,56] This probably means that the source of the increased resistance lies in lung tissue and small airways, rather than large airways. Mean values for respiratory system compliance[43,47,53,55] and resistance[26,30,43,56] are summarized in Table 2.

Table 2
Respiratory System Mechanics and the Work of Breathing in Normals (NL), Obese Subjects (OB) and Obesity Hypoventilation Syndrome (OHS)

Variable	Units	NL	OB	OHS
Crs	(L/cm H_2O)	0.11	0.05	0.06
Rrs	(cm H_2O/L/s)	1.2	4.0	7.8
Work	(J/L)	0.43	0.74	1.64
O_2 cost	(mL/L)	1.1	4.5	10.4
Efficiency	(%)	2.1	0.8	1.0

Crs = respiratory system compliance; Rrs = respiratory system resistance; O_2 cost = mL O_2 consumed by respiratory muscles per liter of ventilation.

Table 3
Pattern of Breathing and Ventilatory Drive in Normals (NL),
Obese Subjects (OB) and Obesity Hypoventilation Syndrome (OHS)

Variable	Units	NLS	OB	OHS
RR	(breath/min)	13.0	17.0	20.0
VT	(mL)	690.0	640.0	490.0
VT	(mL/kg)	9.5	5.2	4.0
DVE/DPCO$_2$	(L/min/torr)	3.1	2.1	0.9
P0.1	(cm H$_2$O)	1.0	1.9	—

RR = respiratory rate; VT = tidal volume; DVE/DPCO$_2$ = slope of ventilatory response to inhaled CO$_2$; P$_{0.1}$ = mouth occlusion pressure.

Work and Energy Cost of Breathing

As a result of increased resistance, a decreased compliance and inspiratory threshold load, the work and energy cost of breathing are increased. Mean values of work per liter of ventilation (expressed in joules per liter) are summarized in Table 2. The work of breathing in simple obesity is 60% higher than normal, versus approximately 250% higher than normal in OHS.

The oxygen cost of breathing represents the oxygen consumed by the respiratory muscles per liter of ventilation. The oxygen cost is a surrogate for the energy cost of breathing. Mean values from several sources[32,43,48,59-61] are presented in Table 3. The energy cost of breathing in simple obesity is four times higher than normal, versus over seven times higher than normal in OHS. Each milliliter of oxygen corresponds to 20.1 J, therefore, efficiency of breathing can be calculated. The values in Table 2 probably underestimate the true efficiency of breathing, but they illustrate the differences between normal and obese subjects. Efficiency is essentially the same in obesity and OHS.

Control of Breathing

Pattern of Breathing

The respiratory rate (RR) of eucapnic morbidly obese subjects is approximately 40% higher than in normal subjects during quiet breathing (Table 3). The duration of inspiration as a fraction of total breath duration (Ti/Ttot) is normal. The tidal volume (Vt) is normal in simple obesity, both at rest and at maximal exercise.[9,23,28,33,35] Patients with OHS have a 25% higher RR and a 25% lower Vt than subjects with simple obesity,[32] but Ti/Ttot remains normal.[28]

When Vt of the obese subject is normalized to BW (Vt, mL/kg) is approximately half normal at rest[9,33,35,39,60,61] and only one-third normal at maximal exercise.[9, 23] It can be calculated from data in Dempsey et al.[9] that the Vt (mL/kg) at maximal exercise is inversely correlated with the percentage of body fat. When related to lean body mass (LBM), Vt is still only 80% of normal at rest and 50% normal at maximal exercise.

Ventilatory Drive

Since patients with OHS, uncomplicated by obstructive airways disease, can attain normal $PaCO_2$ by voluntary hyperventilation,[50] it is likely that ventilatory control is abnormal in OHS. The ventilatory responses to inhalation of carbon dioxide (DVE/DPCO$_2$, Table 3) are generally reduced by approximately 40% in simple obesity and 65% in OHS.[26,28,34,35,47,52] Several reports describe patients who have OHS with normal responses to inhaled CO_2 and markedly reduced ventilatory responses to hypoxic gas mixtures.[25,44] However, the ventilatory response to hypoxia may also be normal or higher than normal in simple obesity, eventhough the obese subjects have a reduced CO_2 response.[35,44] The mean inspiratory flow rate (Vt/Ti) is normal in uncomplicated obesity (Table 3).[28,35,62]

The mouth occlusion pressure ($P_{0.1}$) is about two times normal in obesity (Table 3)[28,35] and it increases normally with CO_2 inhalation.[52] The $P_{0.1}$ in former OHS patients is the same as in obesity,[28,62] but values for $P_{0.1}$ in overt OHS are not available. The mouth occlusion pressure response to CO_2 inhalation is normal in OHS, as compared with two times normal in simple obesity and OSA.[52] Respiratory muscle electrical activity (EMG) responses to inhaled gas mixtures are thought to parallel the mouth occlusion pressure responses. The diaphragm EMG response to inhalation of CO_2 is elevated in uncomplicated obesity, but lies in the normal range in OHS.[47,52]

Sleep Apnea

The prevalence of OSA in simple obesity is approximately 50% in men versus 10% in women, as judged by polysomnography.[63-66] When respiratory disturbances during sleep were monitored by a portable screening technique, 38% of women had some degree of OSA.[67] The higher prevalence of OSA in men is associated with a more upper body fat and higher waist/hip ratios,[13] thicker skin folds,[68] and lower $P_{0.1}$ at rest, as well as lower $P_{0.1}$ and ventilatory responses to carbon dioxide and hypoxia.[65, 68]

The prevalence of sleep apnea in OHS is probably high, but reliable estimates are not available. Sugerman et al.[69] reported on 126 patients with respiratory problems who underwent gastric surgery for weight reduction. This group represented 12.5 % of all patients operated on for obesity from 1980 to 1990. Sixteen patients (94% women) had OHS alone, 45 had OHS and sleep apnea, and 65 had central or OSAs. Thus, 74% of Sugerman's OHS patients also had sleep apnea. Read and Suratt (personal communication) found that 2 of 9 patients with OHS had no apneas, 4 had mild apneas and only 3 had severe central or obstructive apneas. Thus, OSA may not be essential to OHS,[70] but it is widely prevalent and it certainly aggravates hypoxemia and hypercapnia. Conversely, hypercapnia is not a feature of uncomplicated OSA.[52,71 72] When patients with OSA retain CO_2, they usually have diffuse airway obstruction or obesity.[30,31,73]

One important consideration is the rate at or extent to which oxyhemoglobin saturation (SaO_2) falls during an apnea. The principal determinants of the extent of desaturation during an apnea are the lung volume and mixed venous oxyhemoglobin saturation ($SmvO_2$).[74,75] During voluntary breath holding, alveolar PO_2 falls much faster in obese subjects than in normals, and the magnitude of the fall in 15 seconds is correlated with the severity of obesity, the reduction of FRC, the $SmvO_2$, and the oxygen consumption.[75–77]

Respiratory Muscle Strength and Exercise Performance

Respiratory Muscles

Maximal inspiratory and expiratory pressures (PI_{max}, PE_{max}) are normal in eucapnic obese subjects,[4,62,78] but the inspiratory muscles of patients with OHS are approximately 30% weaker than normal (Table 4).[24,28,78] In severely obese subjects the diaphragm may be overstretched, at least in the supine position.[79] This places the diaphragm at a mechanical disadvantage and contributes to the decreased inspiratory strength and efficiency. The MVV, an index of ventilatory en-

Table 4
Exercise Capacity in Normal (NL)
and Obese Subjects (OB)

Variable	Units	NL	OB	OHS
VO2max	(mL/kg/min)	46	28	—
VEmax	(L/min)	93	82	—
MVV	(L/min)	159	129	89
PImax	(cm H_2O)	100	95	60
PEmax	(cm H_2O)	150	125	—

VO_2 = oxygen consumption; VE = minute ventilation; MVV = maximal voluntary ventilation; PImax = maximal inspiratory pressure; PEmax = maximal expiratory pressure.

durance, is approximately 80% of normal in uncomplicated obesity and 55% of normal in OHS (Table 4).[3,32,43,48,53] Little is known about respiratory muscle morphology or contractility in human obesity. A single case report describes fatty infiltration of the diaphragm in a patient with OHS who died in cardiorespiratory failure.[80]

Exercise Capacity

Young adults with uncomplicated obesity have a near normal capacity for physical exercise. Obese subjects at rest consume approximately 25% more oxygen than nonobese subjects.[9,26,33,35,61,76,81] On the cycle ergometer, obese subjects do less external work for a given VO_2 (for example, at 100-W intensity the VO_2 is approximately 20% higher in obese subjects).[9,45,81] Much of the excess VO_2 can be attributed to movement of the leg mass.[82] The maximal cycle ergometer work rate (watts), maximal exercise VO_2, and maximal exercise VE are approximately 90% of normal in young obese subjects.[9,81] On the treadmill, both VE_{max} and VO_{2max} are, again, approximately 20% higher in obese subjects.[10,83] When oxygen consumption at maximal exercise is related to absolute BW, VO_{2max} (mL/kg/min) is lower than normal in the obese subjects and it is inversely correlated with the percentage of body fat.[9,10,83] However, VO_{2max} expressed as mL/kgFFM/min is normal, except in the most in obese subjects.[9,10,83,84] Carbon dioxide production increases as a function of BW, but the rate of increase per kilogram is 40% higher in normal than in obese subjects.[59] After weight loss, the CO_2 production and alveolar ventilation during exercise fall by 12% to 22%.[34]

At the onset of exercise, obese subjects tend to have transient hypoventilation and arterial blood oxyhemoglobin desaturation.[85] Otherwise, the respiratory exchange ratio (VCO_2/VO_2) is normal.[9,33,76] The slopes of the heart rate, blood pressure, VE, Vt, RR, DLCO, and VD/Vt responses of healthy young obese subjects to exercise are very similar to those in young normal subjects.[9,23] At exercise, as at rest, obese subjects breathe faster with a smaller VT.[84,86] The relation between the rate of perceived exertion on the Borg scale and either VO_2 or heart rate, expressed as percent of maximal, is similar to that in normal subjects.[87]

Results in Genetically Obese Animals

In genetically obese (fa/fa) Zucker rats with BWs of 2.3 times of normal animals, FRC and TLC were reduced by 14%.[88] Their lung compliance was normal, but respiratory system compliance was reduced by 24%.[88] The control of breathing is abnormal in genetically obese animals. In the Zucker rat the pattern of breathing was normal, but the ventilatory response to CO_2 was reduced by 39%.[88] In genetically obese (ob/ob) mice the pattern of breathing was normal, but the ventilatory response to hypercapnia was reduced by 30%, even before they became obese, and the ob/ob mice developed tachypnea only after they became obese.[89] Ventilatory responses to hypoxia were normal in both types of obese rat.[88, 89] Thus, genetic determinants influence the ventilatory response to the hypercapnic stimulus, whereas the pattern of breathing may be influenced by the increase in BW.

In one rat model of obesity, the diaphragm had 20% to 30% less muscle mass and 8% to 20% smaller fiber diameter, but a normal distribution of fiber types.[90] In the obese Zucker rat, there were more and thicker type 1 fibers, and the diaphragms of obese animals were 29% thicker and 9% shorter than diaphragms from normal animals.[91] Oxidative capacity, as judged from activity of citrate synthase, was increased in costal and crural diaphragm and parasternal intercostal muscle of obese rats, whereas lactic dehydrogenase activity was lower in these muscles.[92] The percent of type 1 myosin heavy chain was higher, and type 2b myosin heavy chain was lower in diaphragms from obese animals, which is consistent with the hypothesis that obesity causes a fast-to-slow shift in the myosin heavy chain phenotype.[92] The contraction times of diaphragms from obese rats were somewhat faster than normal, the twitch tension normalized to muscle cross-section arca was decreased by 26%, and the maximal tetanic tension was reduced 13% from values in control diaphragms.[91]

Clinical Complications Related to the Respiratory System

Anesthesia and Surgery

Anesthetic management of the obese patient is difficult. Technical problems include transfers from bed to operating table, locating veins and arteries, tracheal intubation, and placement of epidural cannulas. Postoperative positioning and cardiopulmonary monitoring are also difficult. The FRC and PaO_2 often fall further with anesthesia.[93] During mechanical ventilation with a Vt of 13 mL/kg, ideal BW peak airway pressure was approximately 25 cm H_2O, and increasing VT to 22 mL/kg increased peak airway pressure with little effect on PaO_2.[94] Under anesthesia ,and after 5 minutes of 100% oxygen, the time required for SaO_2 to fall to 90% during a deliberately induced apnea was 6 minutes for normal subjects versus less than 3 minutes for obese subjects with BMI 43 kg/m^2.[77] Atelectasis occurs in up to 30% of patients, especially in heavier patients with smaller FRC, but less than 5% in patients with developed pneumonia.[93, 95]

Pulmonary Embolism and Pulmonary Hypertension

Postoperative pulmonary embolism was reported in less than 5% of patients undergoing weight reduction surgery.[93, 95] However, the risk of deep vein thrombosis is increased, the risk of pulmonary embolism is twice as high in obese subjects,[96] and the risk for fatal pulmonary embolism is high in OHS.[97] It is difficult to make a definitive diagnosis of pulmonary embolism in the obese patient because the overlying adipose tissue and small lung volume makes it hard to read ventilation-perfusion scans. Pulmonary hypertension in obesity can result from ventilatory failure,[24] but more importantly, it can result from taking drugs to suppress appetite. In a multicenter European study, the risk of primary pulmonary hypertension was increased 6.3-fold for obese patients who had taken anorexic agents derived from fenfluramine (FFM), and the risk was more than 23-fold for those who had taken the drug for more than 3 months.[98]

Treatment of Morbid Obesity

Weight Loss

The optimal treatment of morbid obesity is weight loss, but this is hard to achieve and often transitory. Obese people underestimate their caloric intake to a substantial degree.[99] Moreover, weight loss induces a reduction in metabolic rate that offsets the effect of dieting.[21, 100] Use of behavior modification and a 1200 kcal/d diet led to 8.5 kg weight loss in 20 weeks, as compared with a 20-kg loss in 12 to 16 weeks with a medically supervised 400 to 800 kcal/d diet.[101] Approximately 60% of the weight loss was maintained for 1 year, but patients returned to their original weight in 5 years.[101] With a 1000 kcal/d diet alone, total weight loss was 7.8 kg in 12 weeks, which included 1.2 kg of FFM.[102] When the diet was combined with exercise the total weight loss was 10.3 kg, with no loss of FFM.[102]

Current surgical procedures for weight loss include vertical banded gastroplasty, Roux-en-Y gastic bypass, and panniculectomy. Patients whose initial weight was 172 kg lost 19% of their BW after panniculectomy, but the long-term weight loss was not recorded.[95] Patients undergoing gastric bypass lost 50% to 75% of their excess weight within 2 years and maintained more than 80% of the weight loss for 5 to 10 years.[103–105] Patients who underwent vertical gastric banding lost 50% to 60% of their excess weight by 2 years, while some maintained most of the weight loss for 4 to 7 years, however, approximately 30% returned to or above their initial weight by 10 years.[103,105,106] After gastrostomy alone, patients who weighed 139 kg lost 19% of their BW in 1 year, but regained 67% of this by 10 years.[107] After gastric bypass, patients who weighed 136 kg lost 28% of their BW by 1 year and regained only 25% by 10 years.[107] The magnitude and duration of benefits of gastric surgery are the same for patients with OHS and/or sleep apnea as they are for simple obesity.[69,108]

Effects on Pulmonary Function and Gas Exchange

In simple obesity, pulmonary function and arterial blood gases improved after weight loss induced by small bowel bypass or gastric surgery,[34,36,44,49,109–111] or low calorie diets.[26,27,29,37] The most striking change in pulmonary function was the increase in ERV. For example, weight loss of 40 kg reduced BMI from 50 to 37 kg/m^2, with a 75% increase in ERV, a 25% increase in RV and FRC, and a 10% increase in MVV. Weight loss is associated with a small, but statistically significant, increase in VC,[37] but there was little change in FEV_1/FVC, TLC or compliance, and some patients developed mild respiratory muscle weakness.[112] Weight loss sometimes increased PaO_2 in eucapnic obese patients,[27,34,36,113] especially if weight loss reduced BW to less than 130% of ideal.[27] There was a slight reduction in DLCO.[3,36] The DVE/$DPaCO_2$ fell slightly, but not significantly, after weight loss.[26,34,44,109] Ketosis associated with acute fasting had no effect on DVE/$DPaCO_2$ or any other variable in uncomplicated obesity.[114] Weight loss was associated with a substantial reduction in CO_2 production during exercise.[34]

Obesity-Hypoventilation Syndrome

The effects of weight loss on pulmonary function are far more striking in OHS. With an average weight loss of 35 kg, VC increased from 53% to 84%, predicted; ERV increased from 33% to 59%, predicted; and FRC increased from 59% to 75%, predicted. Concomitantly, $PaCO_2$ fell and PaO_2 rose, each by 15 mm Hg.[24,43,49] MVV often increased significantly with weight loss.[24] In one patient's weight loss, the oxygen cost of breathing fell from 9 times normal to normal, and the diaphragm EMG response to inhaled CO_2 increased more than 10-fold.[24] In OHS ketosis induced by fasting increased the DVE/$DPaCO_2$, with the increase being proportional to the degree of ketosis.[114]

Ventilatory Failure

Weight loss is the most important component of the long-term management of ventilatory failure. When patients with OHS can lose weight, their ventilatory function improves substantially. As BW decreases, $PaCO_2$ also decreases, while VC increases.[24] Patients with OHS and OSA experience fewer and less severe nocturnal desaturations, as well as improvement in daytime PaO_2 and $PaCO_2$.[63,71,72]

Mechanical ventilation with a negative pressure body respirator suppresses diaphragmatic activity in patients with OHS and other diseases with ventilatory failure.[115] This allows patients to be ventilated and oxygenated without worrying about worsening hypercapnia,[116] and it improves sleep in some patients.[117] Unfortunately, negative pressure ventilation may induce OSA in patients with neuromuscular, chest wall, and obstructive airways diseases.[118,119] Oxygen therapy tends to aggravate sleep apnea, but nasal continuous positive airway pressure (CPAP) added to negative pressure ventilation alleviates apnea.[120]

Noninvasive mechanical ventilation may also be provided by positive pressure ventilation by nose mask. Unlike negative pressure ventilation, positive pressure ventilation improves sleep substantially.[121] Hill[122] suggests that the principal benefit of nocturnal nasal ventilation is relief of hypoventilation. In six patients who had both OHS and OSA, 24 hours of continuous CPAP raised pH from 7.23 to 7.35, lowered $PaCO_2$ from 80 to 64 mm Hg, and increased PaO_2 from 55 to 69 mm Hg.[123] In 13 patients with OHS and OSA, who failed initial CPAP, nocturnal nasal positive pressure ventilation increased PaO_2 from 50 to 66 mm Hg and lowered $PaCO_2$ from 62 to 46 mm Hg; they were subsequently maintained on CPAP.[124]

The complications from nose mask CPAP or ventilation include erosion of skin, especially over the bridge of the nose,[125] and exacerbation of nasal stuffiness or sinusitis.[126] It is possible that delivery of CPAP or positive pressure ventilation via the mouth would be better for chronic use. This is accomplished by using a lip seal device to prevent leaks at the mouth.[127,128]

Case Presentation

A 64-year-old obese housekeeper was admitted to a hospital with chest tightness and dyspnea at rest. She had been heavy for many years, then lost over 40 kg a year prior to admission, but recently gained it back. In the 1 month prior to admission she had progressive exertional dyspnea, chest and abdominal tightness, increasing abdominal girth, and swelling of the legs.

The physical examination revealed blood pressure 142/100, heart rate 124, RR 36, and BW 144 kg (225% ideal). There were wheezes and rales over the lower one-third of chest bilaterally, tachycardia with S_4 gallop, and jugular venous distention. The abdomen was obese and there was 3+ pitting edema of the legs. Initial arterial blood gas analysis showed a pH of 7.29, $PaCO_2$ of 75 mm Hg, and HCO_3^- 32 mEq/L. The PaO_2 was 43 mm Hg, the SaO_2 was 78% on room air, and the hematocrit was 55%. The ECG showed atrial flutter with 2:1 AV conduction. The chest x-ray showed poor inspiration, and a ventilation/perfusion scan was read as high probability for pulmonary embolism.

She was anticoagulated with heparin. Somnolence worsened on treatment with digoxin and procainamide without supplemental oxygen. On the third hospital day, the pH was 7.22, $PaCO_2$ was 85 mm Hg, and HCO_3^- 34 mEq/L; PaO_2 was 40 mm Hg and SaO_2 was 75% on room air. She was given metoprolol and intravenous diltiazem for the atrial flutter, but she became hypotensive and was transferred to medical intensive care unit where she was intubated, mechanically ventilated, and oxygenated. The SaO_2 was maintained above 90% and $PaCO_2$ was lowered slowly to less than 50 mm Hg. After stabilization, she received furosemide for diuresis, acetazolamide to promote HCO_3^- excretion, and later spironolactone. Her total weight loss exceeded 20 kg. She was cardioverted on the fifth hospital day, and extubated on the eighth hospital day.

She then started BiPAP ventilation plus oxygen at 2 L/min. She switched to nocturnal BiPAP on the 10th hospital day and was discharged home on the 13th hospital day. Medications were digoxin, spironolactone, BiPAP, and oxygen at 2 L/min with BiPAP, as well as by nasal cannula. On discharge the pH was 7.40, $PaCO_2$ was 59 mm Hg, HCO_3^- was 35 mEq/L; PaO_2 was 47 mm Hg and SaO_2 was 83% on room air. A polysomnography study performed after discharge showed central apneas and hypopneas with desaturation to 65% without CPAP, and marked improvement with CPAP. In the subsequent 3 years, she has not been rehospitalized.

This case illustrates several important therapeutic points. First, it is absolutely necessary to maintain adequate oxygenation. Trying to treat the arrhythmia without oxygenation led to hypotension, which was rapidly reversible with intubation, mechanical ventilation, and oxygenation. Second, mechanical ventilatory support coupled with diuretics that promoted bicarbonate excretion and inhibition of aldosterone facilitated weight loss and normalization of pH and $PaCO_2$. Third, hypoxemia was relatively resistant to therapy. Fourth, this patient did not have OSA, but she needed CPAP to relieve hypopneas.

Summary

Morbid obesity without hypoventilation is characterized by marked increases in BW and BMI, mostly from excess fat, but also from an increase in fat-free mass. Obesity reduces the ERV and to a lesser extent the FRC. The VC and TLC are normal, except in very severe obesity. Hypoxemia results from overperfusion of dependent lung zones, which are very poorly ventilated, and owe to the fall in ERV. The largest improvements with weight loss are restoration of the ERV and PaO_2 toward, but not entirely, to normal.

In simple obesity, respiratory resistance is three times normal and respiratory system compliance is half normal. Obesity doubles the work of breathing and quadruples the energy cost of breathing. To meet these demands, ventilatory drive is doubled and the pattern of breathing shifts to a higher RR and a smaller VT. Inspiratory muscle strength is well preserved, but the MVV is somewhat reduced. Obese subjects have a relatively normal capacity for physical exercise. However, they have to expend more work during treadmill or bicycle exercise becuase of the excess load imposed by the mass of their body or legs, and impaired pulmonary gas exchange limits the available energy supply to a mild degree.

BW in the OHS is the same as in uncomplicated morbid obesity. The respiratory abnormalities of uncomplicated morbid obesity are present, but more severe, in OHS. The VC is reduced by one-third and the ERV is reduced by two-thirds. Respiratory resistance is eight times normal, the work of breathing is four times normal, and the oxygen cost of breathing is nine times normal. Moreover, in OHS the inspiratory muscles are somewhat weak and ventilatory drive is not increased to meet the increased work of breathing. The RR is higher and the VT is smaller in OHS than in uncomplicated obesity.

Increases in ventilatory drive and respiratory muscle contractile effort are required to maintain ventilation in the presence of the increased ventilatory load of obesity. When the ventilatory load is more severe, and the respiratory muscles are weaker, a merely normal ventilatory drive is inadequate. Thus, it is likely that the ventilatory characteristics of OHS suffice to explain the CO_2 retention, without having to invoke OSA.

When present, central sleep apneas or OSAs only make matters worse. OSA is approximately five times as common in obese men as in obese women, and the increased prevalence of OSA in men appears to be related to a more central (visceral) distribution of fat and lower sensitivity to inhaled CO_2. Many, but not all, patients with OHS have severe OSA.

Key elements in treatment of OHS are oxygenation, relief of upper airway obstruction when present, and weight loss. The roles of CPAP and mechanical ventilation are to prevent inspiratory closure of upper airways, permit oxygenation without development of respiratory acidosis, and correct acute respiratory acidosis. Providing CPAP or ventilation by nose mask is often helpful, but use of other modalities such as the lip seal might work as well. Weight loss is associated with increased VC, lowering of $PaCO_2$, and lessening of sleep-related apneas and hypopneas. Hypoxia is relatively resistant to treatment if there is severe shunting through nonventilated regions.

References

1. Metropolitan Life Insurance Company: *Stat Bull* 40:1–4, 1959.
2. Seltzer F: Measurement of overweight. *Stat Bull* 65:20–23, 1984.
3. Ray CS, Sue DY, Bray G, et al: Effects of obesity on respiratory function. *Am Rev Respir Dis* 128:501–506, 1984.
4. Kelly TM, Jensen RL, Elliott CG, et al: Maximum respiratory pressures in morbidly obese subjects. *Respiration* 54:73–77, 1988.
5. Fung KP, Lee J, Lau SP, et al: Properties and clinical implications of body mass index. *Arch Dis Child* 65:516–519, 1990.
6. Pierson RNJ, Wang J, Heymsfield SB, et al: Measuring body fat: Calibrating the rulers. Intermethod comparison in 389 normal Caucasian subjects. *Am J Physiol* 261:E103-E108, 1991.
7. Morse WI, Soeldner JS: The composition of adipose tissue and the nonadipose body of obese and nonobese men. *Metabolism* 12:99–107, 1963.
8. Morse WI, Soeldner JS: The nonadipose body mass of obese women: Evidence of increased muscularity. *Can Med Assoc J* 90:723–725, 1964
9. Dempsey JA, Reddan W, Balke B, et al: Work capacity determinants and physiologic cost of weight-supported work in obesity. *J Appl Physiol* 21:1815–1820, 1966.
10. Kollias J, Boileau RA, Bartlett HL, et al: Pulmonary function and physical conditioning in lean and obese subjects. *Arch Environ Health* 25:146–150, 1972.
11. Morgan NG, Durnin JVGA: The effect of 6 weeks of overfeeding on the body weight, body composition, and energy metabolism of young men. *Am J Clin Nutr* 33:978–988, 1980.
12. Levinson PD, McGarvey ST, Carlisle CC, et al: Adiposity and cardiovascular risk factors in men with obstructive sleep apnea. *Chest* 103:1336–1342, 1993.
13. Millman RP, Carlisle CC, McGarvey ST, et al: Body fat distribution and sleep apnea severity in women. *Chest* 107:362–366, 1995.
14. Collins LC, Hoberty PD, Walker JF, et al: The effect of body fat distribution on pulmonary function tests. *Chest* 107:1298–1302, 1995.
15. Suzuki R, Watanabe S, Hirai Y, et al: Abdominal wall fat index, estimated by ultrasonography, for assessment of the ratio of visceral fat to subcutaneous fat in the abdomen. *Am J Med* 95:309–314, 1993.
16. Muls E, Vyrens C, Michels A, et al: The effect of abdominal fat distribution on the respiratory system in non-smoking obese women. *International J Obesity* 14:136(Abstract), 1990.
17. Busetto L, Baggio MB, Zurlo F, et al: Assessment of abdominal fat distribution in obese patients: Anthropometry *versus* computerized tomography. *Int J Obes* 16:731–736, 1992.
18. Sobol W, Rossner S, Hinson B, et al: Evaluation of a new magnetic resonance imaging method for quantitating adipose tissue areas. *Int J Obes* 15:589–599, 1991.
19. Ross R, Shaw KD, Rissanen J, et al: Sex differences in lean and adipose tissue distribution by magnetic resonance imaging: Anthropometric relationships. *Am J Clin Nutr* 59:1277–1285, 1994.

20. Verga S, Buscemi C, Caimi G: Resting energy expenditure and body composition in morbidly obese, obese and control subjects. *Acta Diabetol Lat* 31:47–51, 1994.
21. Leibel RL, Rosenbaum M, Hirsch J: Changes in energy expenditure resulting from altered body weight. *N Engl J Med* 332:621–628, 1995.
22. Gray DS, Fujioka K: Use of relative weight and body mass index for the determination of adiposity. *J Clin Epidemiol* 44:545–550, 1991.
23. Dempsey JA, Reddan W, Rankin J, et al: Alveolar-arterial gas exchange during muscular work in obesity. *J Appl Physiol* 21:1807–1814, 1966.
24. Rochester DF, Enson Y: Current concepts in the pathogenesis of the obesity-hypoventilation syndrome. *Am J Med* 57:402–420, 1974.
25. Zwillich CW, Sutton FD, Pierson DJ, et al: Decreased hypoxic ventilatory drive in the obesity-hypoventilation syndrome. *Am J Med* 59:343–348, 1975.
26. Emirgil C, Sobol BJ: The effects of weight reduction on pulmonary function and the sensitivity of the respiratory center in obesity. *Am Rev Respir Dis* 108:831–842, 1973.
27. Farebrother MJB, McHardy GJR, Munro JF: Relation between pulmonary gas exchange and volume before and after substantial weight loss in obese subjects. *Br Med J* 3:391–393. 1974.
28. Sampson MG, Grassino A: Neuromechanical properties in obese patients during carbon dioxide rebreathing. *Am J Med* 75:81–90, 1983.
29. Smith PL, Gold AR, Meyers DA, et al: Weight loss in mildly to moderately obese patients with obstructive sleep apnea. *Ann Intern Med* 103:850–855, 1985.
30. Bradley TD, Rutherford R, Lue F, et al: Role of diffuse airway obstruction in the hypercapnia of obstructive sleep apnea. *Am Rev Respir Dis* 134: 920–924, 1986.
31. Leech J, Onal E, Baer P, et al: Determinants of hypercapnia in occlusive sleep apnea syndrome. *Chest* 92:807–813, 1987.
32. Kaufman BJ, Ferguson MH, Cherniack RM: Hypoventilation in obesity. *J Clin Invest* 38:500–507, 1959.
33. Barrera F, Hillyer P, Asciano G, et al: The distribution of ventilation, diffusion, and blood flow in obese patients with normal and abnormal blood gases. *Am Rev Respir Dis* 108:819–830, 1973.
34. Jacobsen E, Dano P, Skovsted P: Respiratory function before and after weight loss following intestinal shunt operation for obesity. *Scand J Respir Dis* 55:332–339, 1974.
35. Burki NK, Baker RW: Ventilatory regulation in eucapnic morbid obesity. *Am Rev Respir Dis* 129:538–543, 1984.
36. Thomas PS, Cowen ERT, Hulands G, et al: Respiratory function in the morbidly obese before and after weight loss. *Thorax* 44:382–386, 1989.
37. Hakala K, Mustajoki P, Aittomaki J, et al: Effect of weight loss and body position on pulmonary function and gas exchange abnormalities in morbid obesity. *International J Obesity* 19:343–346, 1995.
38. Holley H, Milic-Emili J, Becklake M, et al: Regional distribution of pulmonary ventilation and perfusion in obesity. *J Clin Invest* 46:475–481, 1967.
39. Barrera F, Reidenberg MM, Winters WL, et al: Ventilation-perfusion relationships in the obese patient. *J Appl Physiol* 26:420–426, 1969.

40. Hurewitz AN, Susskind H, Harold WH: Obesity alters regional ventilation in lateral decubitus position. *J Appl Physiol* 59:774–783, 1985.
41. Douglas FG, Chong PY: Influence of obesity on peripheral airways patency. *J Appl Physiol* 33:559–563, 1972.
42. Prefaut C, Monnier L, Ramonatxo M, et al: Influence de la posture et de la fermeture des voies ariennes sur les echanges respiratoires du sujet obese. *Bull Eur Physiopath Resp* 14:249–263, 1978.
43. Sharp JT, Henry JP, Sweany SK, et al: The total work of breathing in normal and obese men. *J Clin Invest* 43:728–739, 1964.
44. Kronenberg RS, Gabel RA, Severinghaus JW: Normal chemoreceptor function in obesity before and after ileal bypass surgery to force weight reduction. *Am J Med* 59:349–353, 1975.
45. Bray GA, Whipp BJ, Koyal SN, et al: Some respiratory and metabolic effects of exercise in moderately obese men. *Metabolism* 26:403–412, 1977.
46. Knochel JP: Neuromuscular manifestations of electrolyte disorders. *Am J Med* 72:521–535, 1982.
47. Lourenco RV: Diaphragm activity in obesity. *J Clin Invest* 48:1609–1614, 1969.
48. Fritts HW Jr, Filler J, Fishman AP, et al: The efficiency of ventilation during voluntary hyperpnea: Studies in normal subjects and in dyspneic patients with either chronic pulmonary emphysema or obesity. *J Clin Invest* 38:1339–1348, 1959.
49. Sugerman HJ, Fairman RP, Baron PL, et al: Gastric surgery for respiratory insufficiency of obesity. *Chest* 90:81–86, 1986.
50. Leech J, Onal E, Aronson R, et al: Voluntary hyperventilation in obesity hypoventilation. *Chest* 100:1334–1338, 1991.
51. Jenkins SC, Moxham J: The effects of mild obesity on lung function. *Respir Med* 85:309–311, 1991.
52. Lopata M, Onal E: Mass loading, sleep apnea, and the pathogenesis of obesity hypoventilation. *Am Rev Respir Dis* 126:640–645, 1982.
53. Naimark A, Cherniack RM: Compliance of the respiratory system and its components in health and obesity. *J Appl Physiol* 15:377–382, 1960.
54. Pelosi P, Croci M, Ravagnaan I, et al: Total respiratory system, lung, and chest wall mechanics in sedated-paralyzed postoperative morbidly obese patients. *Chest* 109:144–151, 1996.
55. Suratt PM, Wilhoit S, Hsiao H, et al: Compliance of chest wall in obese subjects. *J Appl Physiol* 57:403–407, 1984.
56. Zerah F, Harf A, Perlemuter L, et al: Effects of obesity on respiratory resistance. *Chest* 103:1470–1476, 1993.
57. Rubinstein I, Zamel N, DuBarry RPT, et al: Airflow limitation in morbidly obese, nonsmoking men. *Ann Intern Med* 112:828–832, 1990.
58. Yap JCH, Watson RA, Gilbey S, et al: Effects of posture on respiratory mechanics in obesity. *J Appl Physiol* 79:1199–1205, 1995.
59. Gilbert R, Sipple JH, Auchincloss JH: Respiratory control and work of breathing in obese subjects. *J Appl Physiol* 16:21–26, 1961.
60. Cherniack RM, Guenter CA: The efficiency of the respiratory muscles in obesity. *Can J Biochem Physiol* 39:1215–1222, 1961.
61. Bosman AR, Goldman HI: The oxygen cost and work of breathing in normal and obese subjects. *S Afr J Lab Clin Med* 7:62–67, 1961.

62. Sampson MG, Grassino AE: Load compensation in obese patients during quiet tidal breathing. *J Appl Physiol* 55:1269–1276, 1983.
63. Rajala R, Partinen M, Sane T, et al: Obstructive sleep apnea syndrome in morbidly obese patients. *J Intern Med* 230:125–129, 1991.
64. Vgontzas AN, Tan TL, Bixler EO, et al: Sleep apnea and sleep disruption in obese patients. *Arch Intern Med* 154:1705–1711, 1994.
65. Kunitomo F, Kimura H, Tatsumi K, et al: Sex differences in awake ventilatory drive and abnormal breathing during sleep in eucapnic obesity. *Chest* 93:968–976, 1988.
66. Broussole C, Piperno D, Gormand F, et al: [Sleep apnea syndrome in obese patients: are there any predictive factors?] *Revue de Medecine Interne* 15:161–165, 1994.
67. Richman RM, Elliott LM, Burns CM, et al: The prevalence of obstructive sleep apnea in an obese female population. *Int J Obes* 18:173–177, 1994.
68. Gold AR, Schwartz AR, Wise RA, et al: Pulmonary function and respiratory chemosensitivity in moderately obese patients with sleep apnea. *Chest* 103:1325–1329, 1993.
69. Sugerman HJ, Fairman RP, Wolfe L, et al: Long-term effects of gastric surgery for treating respiratory insufficiency of obesity. *Am J Clin Nutr* 55:597S–601S, 1992.
70. Rapoport DM, Garay SM, Epstein H, et al: Hypercapnia in the obstructive sleep apnea syndrome. A reevaluation of the "Pickwickian syndrome." *Chest* 89:627–635, 1986.
71. Harman EM, Wynne JY, Block AJ: The effect of weight loss on sleep-disordered breathing and oxygen desaturation in morbidly obese men. *Chest* 82:291–294, 1981.
72. Suratt PM, McTier RF, Findley LJ, et al: Changes in breathing and the pharynx after weight loss in obstructive sleep apnea. *Chest* 92:631–637, 1987.
73. Krieger J, Sforza E, Apprill M, et al: Pulmonary hypertension, hypoxemia, and hypercapnia in obstructive sleep apnea patients. *Chest* 96:729–737, 1989.
74. Findley LJ, Ries AL, Tisi GM, et al: Hypoxemia during apnea in normal subjects: Mechanisms and impact of lung volume. *J Appl Physiol* 55:1777–1783, 1983.
75. Fletcher EC, Costarangos C, Miller T: The rate of fall of arterial oxyhemoglobin saturation in obstructive sleep apnea. *Chest* 96:717–722, 1989.
76. Hurewitz A, Sampson MG: Voluntary breath holding in the obese. *J Appl Physiol* 62:2371–2376, 1987.
77. Jense HG, Dubin SA, Silverstein PI, et al: Effect of obesity on safe duration of apnea in anesthetized patients. *Anesth Analg* 72:89–93, 1991.
78. Rochester DF, Arora NS: Respiratory failure from obesity. In Mancini M, Lewis B, Contaldo F (eds): *Medical Complications of Obesity.* Academic Press, New York, 1979, pp. 183–190.
79. Sharp JT, Druz WS, Kondragunta VR: Diaphragmatic responses to body position changes in obese patients with obstructive sleep apnea. *Am Rev Respir Dis* 133:32–37, 1986.
80. Fadell EJ, Richman AD, Ward WW, et al: Fatty infiltration of respiratory muscles in the Pickwickian syndrome. *N Engl J Med* 266:861–863, 1962.

81. Salvadori A, Fanari P, Mazza P, et al: Work capacity and cardiopulmonary adaptation of the obese subject during exercise testing. *Chest* 101:674–679, 1992.
82. Whipp BJ, Davis JA: The ventilatory stress of exercise in obesity. *Am Rev Respir Dis* 129:S90-S92, 1984.
83. Babb TG, Korzick D, Meador M, et al: Ventilatory response of moderately obese women to submaximal exercise. *Int J Obes* 15:59–65, 1991.
84. Sakamoto S, Ishikawa K, Senda S, et al: The effect of obesity on ventilatory response and anaerobic threshold during exercise. *J Med Sys* 17:227–231, 1993.
85. Auchincloss JH Jr, Sipple J, Gilbert R: Effect of obesity on ventilatory adjustment to exercise. *J Appl Physiol* 18:19–24, 1963.
86. Salvadori A, Fanari P, Mazza P, et al: Breathing pattern during and after maximal exercise testing in young untrained subjects and obese patients. *Respiration* 60:162–169, 1993.
87. Jakicic JM, Pronk NP, Jawad AF, et al: Prescription of exercise intensity for the obese patient: The relationship between heart rate, VO_2 and perceived exertion. *Int J Obes* 19:382–387, 1995.
88. Farkas GA, Schlenker EH: Pulmonary ventilation and mechanics in morbidly obese Zucker rats. *Am J Respir Crit Care Med* 150:356–362, 1994.
89. Tankersley C, Kleeberger S, Russ B, et al: Modified control of breathing in genetically obese (ob/ob) mice. *J Appl Physiol* 81:716–723, 1996.
90. Burbach JA, Schlenker EH, Goldman M: Characterization of muscles from aspartic acid obese rats. *Am J Physiol* 249:R106-R110, 1985.
91. Farkas GA, Gosselin LE, Zhan W-Z, et al: Histochemical and mechanical properties of diaphragm muscle in morbidly obese Zucker rats. *J Appl Physiol* 77:2250–2259, 1994.
92. Powers SK, Farkas GA, Demirel H, et al: Effects of aging and obesity on respiratory muscle phenotype in Zucker rats. *J Appl Physiol* 81:1347–1354, 1996.
93. Fox GS, Whalley DG, Bevan DR: Anesthesia for the morbidly obese: Experience with 110 patients. *Br J Anaesth* 53:811–816, 1981.
94. Bardoczky GI, Yernault JC, Houben JJ, et al: Large tidal volume ventilation does not improve oxygenation in morbidly obese patients during anesthesia. *Anesth Analg* 81:385–388, 1995.
95. Matory WE Jr, O'Sullivan J, Fudem G, et al: Abdominal surgery in patients with severe morbid obesity. *Plast Reconstr Surg* 94:976–987, 1994.
96. Shenkman Z, Shir Y, Brodsky JB: Perioperative management of the obese patient. *Br J Anaesth* 70:349–359, 1993.
97. Miller A, Granada M: In-hospital mortality in the Pickwickian syndrome. *Am J Med* 56:144–150, 1974.
98. Abenhaim L, Moride Y, Brenot F, et al: Appetite suppressant drugs and the risk of primary pulmonary hypertension. *N Engl J Med* 335:609–616, 1996.
99. Lichtman SW, Pisarska K, Berman ER, et al: Discrepancy between self-reported and actual caloric intake and exercise in obese subjects. *N Engl J Med* 327:1893–1898, 1992.
100. Valtuena S, Blanch S, Barenys M, et al: Changes in body composition and resting energy expenditure after rapid weight loss: Is there an energy-metabolism adaptation in obese patients? *Int J Obes* 19:119–125, 1995.

101. Wadden TA: Treatment of obesity by moderate and severe caloric restriction. Results of clinical research trials. *Ann Intern Med* 119:688–693, 1993.
102. Svendsen OL, Hassager C, Christiansen C: Effect of an energy-restrictive diet, with or without exercise, on lean tissue mass, resting metabolic rate, cardiovascular risk factors, and bone overweight postmenopausal women. *Am J Med* 95:131–140, 1993.
103. Sugerman HJ, Kellum JM, Engle KM, et al: Gastric bypass for treating severe obesity. *Am J Clin Nutr* 55:560S-566S, 1992.
104. Pories WJ, MacDonald KGJ, Morgan EJ, et al: Surgical treatment of obesity and its effect on diabetes. *Am J Clin Nutr* 55:582S-585S, 1992.
105. Brolin RE: Critical analysis of results: Weight loss and quality of data. *Am J Clin Nutr* 55(2 Suppl):577S-581S, 1992.
106. Ramsey-Stewart G: Vertical banded gastroplasty for morbid obesity: Weight loss at short and long-term follow up. *Aust NZ J Surg* 65:4–7, 1995.
107. Wolfel R, Gunther K, Rumenapf G, et al: Weight reduction after gastric bypass and horizontal gastroplasty for morbid obesity. *Eur J Surg* 160:219–225, 1994.
108. Charuzi I, Lavie P, Peiser J, et al: Bariatric surgery in morbidly obese sleep-apnea patients: Short- and long-term follow-up. *Am J Clin Nutr* 55:594S-596S, 1992.
109. Soderberg M, Thomson D, White T: Respiration, circulation and anesthetic management in obesity. Investigation before and after jejunoileal bypass. *Acta Anaesth Scand* 21:55–61, 1977.
110. Stalnecker MC, Suratt PM, Chandler JG: Changes in respiratory function following small bowel bypass for obesity. *Surgery* 99:645–651, 1980.
111. Chapman KR, Himal HS, Rebuck AS: Ventilatory responses to hypercapnia and hypoxia in patients with eucapnic morbid obesity before and after weight loss. *Clin Sci* 78:541–545, 1990.
112. Wadstrom C, Muller-Suur R, Backman L: Influence of excessive weight loss on respiratory function. A study of obese patients following gastroplasty. *Eur J Surg* 157:341–346, 1991.
113. Chan CS, Grunstein RR, Bye PTP, et al: Obstructive sleep apnea with severe chronic airflow limitation. *Am Rev Respir Dis* 140:1274–1278, 1989.
114. Fried PI, McClean PA, Phillipson EA, et al: Effect of ketosis on respiratory sensitivity to carbon dioxide in obesity. *N Engl J Med* 294:1081–1086, 1976.
115. Rochester DF, Braun NT, Laine S: Diaphragmatic energy expenditure in chronic respiratory failure. *Am J Med* 63:223–232, 1977.
116. Sauret JM, Guitart AC, Rodriguez-Frojan G, et al: Intermittent short-term negative pressure ventilation and increased oxygenation in COPD patients with severe hypercapnic respiratory failure. *Chest* 100:455–459, 1991.
117. Goldstein RS, Molotiu N, Skrastins R, et al: Assisting ventilation in respiratory failure by negative pressure ventilation and by rocking bed. *Chest* 92:470–474, 1987.
118. Bach JR, Penek J: Obstructive sleep apnea complicating negative-pressure ventilatory support in patients with chronic paralytic/restrictive ventilatory dysfunction. *Chest* 99:1386–1393, 1991.

119. Levy RD, Cosio MG, Gibbons L, et al: Induction of sleep apnea with negative pressure ventilation in patients with chronic obstructive lung disease. *Thorax* 47:612–615, 1992.
120. Hill NS, Redline S, Carskadon MA, et al: Sleep-disordered breathing in patients with Duchenne muscular dystrophy using negative pressure ventilators. *Chest* 102:1656–1662, 1992.
121. Waldhorn RE: Nocturnal nasal intermittent positive pressure ventilation with bi-level positive airway pressure (BiPAP) in respiratory failure. *Chest* 101:516–521, 1992.
122. Hill NS: Noninvasive ventilation. Does it work, for whom, how? *Am Rev Respir Dis* 147:1050–1055, 1993.
123. Shivaram U, Cash ME, Beal A: Nasal continuous positive airway pressure in decompensated hypercapnic respiratory failure as a complication of sleep apnea. *Chest* 104:770–774, 1993.
124. Piper AJ, Sullivan CE: Effects of short-term NIPPV in the treatment of patients with severe obstructive sleep apnea and hypercapnia. *Chest* 105:434–440, 1994.
125. Gay PC, Patel AM, Viggiano RW, et al: Nocturnal nasal ventilation for treatment of patients with hypercapnic respiratory failure. *Mayo Clin Proc* 66:695–703, 1991.
126. Marino W: Intermittent volume cycled mechanical ventilation via nasal mask in patients with respiratory failure due to COPD. *Chest* 99:681–684, 1991.
127. Curran FJ, Colbert AP: Ventilator management in Duchenne muscular dystrophy and postpoliomyelitis syndrome: Twelve years' experience. *Arch Phys Med Rehab* 70:180–185, 1989.
128. Bach JR, Alba AS: Noninvasive options for ventilatory support of the traumatic high level quadriplegic patient. *Chest* 98:613–619, 1990.

Chapter 9

Pathogenesis and Clinical Manifestations of Obesity Cardiomyopathy

James K. Alexander, MD
Martin A. Alpert, MD

The combined effects of increased left ventricular (LV) volume and hypertrophy with associated alterations in LV pressure volume relations, increments in blood volume, and high cardiac output may lead to pulmonary congestion at rest or during exercise in morbidly obese subjects.[1,2] Increased work of breathing,[3] increased ventilation,[4] and relative increase in work of ambulation[5] further exacerbate the effect of circulatory factors in the limitation of exercise tolerance and genesis of exertional dyspnea. Signs and symptoms of circulatory congestion do not usually develop unless body weight is approximately 135 kg, relative weight is 175% to 200%, or body mass index (BMI) is greater than 40 kg/m². Most of the subjects with congestion have maintained these levels of obesity for usually 10 years or longer. Often there is a history of recent weight gain preceding development of increasing dyspnea and leg edema, orthopnea, and abdominal swelling. Development of the congestive state probably occurs in about 10% of these extremely obese subjects.[6] The precipitating mechanisms have not been well defined. It is tempting to hypothesize that they may be the same amount of patients with other high cardiac output states, such as arteriovenous fistula and fistula heart disease. Acute pulmonary edema is uncommon. Regression or progression of the congestive state, corresponding to periods of weight loss or gain, may occur over a number of years. There appears to be a roughly linear correlation between LV wall thickness to

From: Alpert MA, and Alexander JK, (eds). *The Heart and Lung in Obesity.* Armonk, NY: Futura Publishing Company, Inc., © 1998.

cavity radius, an index of wall stress, and LV systolic performance, as indicated by echocardiographically measured LV minor axis shortening fraction (Figure 1). It has been suggested that the increased LV wall stress in some subjects results from "inadequate" myocardial hypertrophy, and that long-term increase in wall stress leads to myocardial decompensation and congestive heart failure (CHF).[7,8] Thus, the clinical presentation may reflect two possible physiological sequences associated with preservation or depression of LV systolic function. Table 1 illustrates data on hemodynamic parameters and LV function in a 36-year-old man with severe pulmonary congestive symptoms, who weighed 200 kg at the time of cardiac catheterization. Body oxygen consumption and cardiac output at rest are both markedly elevated, with a normal arteriovenous oxygen difference. Abnormally high LV diastolic pressure is accompanied by pulmonary hypertension in the presence of normal LV systolic and aortic pressures. Angiographic study demonstrated normal mean LV circumferential fiber shortening rate and ejection fraction. Although LV end-diastolic volume per square me-

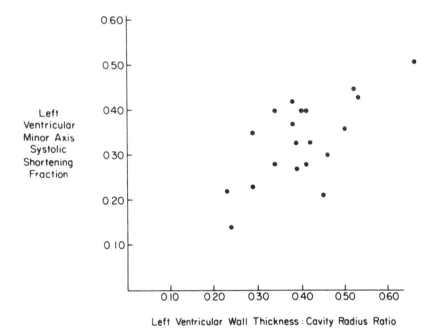

Figure 1. Relation between LV minor axis systolic shortening fraction and ratio of wall thickness to cavity radius in 20 morbidly obese subjects. The ratio tends to fall with worsening of LV function as indicated by reduction in shortening fraction. (Reproduced from Reference 14 with permission.)

Table 1
Circulatory Dynamics and Left Ventricular Function in a
Very Obese Man with High Output Circulatory Congestive State

VO_2 mL/min	405	VCF (circum/sec)	1.75
A-VO_2 (vol %)	3.5	EF (%)	0.78
Q (L/mn)	11.6	LVEDV (mL)	215
PAP (mmHg)	52/19	LVEDC (10^{-2}/mmHg)	1.6
LVP (mmHg)	135/17	LVEDWT (cm)	1.4
AoP (mmHg)	135/85		

VO_2 = oxygen consumption; A-VO_2 = arteriovenous oxygen difference; Q = cardiac output; PAP = pulmonary artery pressure, systolic/diastolic; LVP = left ventricular pressure, systolic/end-diastolic; AoP = aortic pressure, systolic/diastolic; VCF = mean circumferential, fiber shortening rate; EF = left ventricular ejection fraction; LVEDV = left ventricular end-diastolic volume; LVEDC = left ventricular end-diastolic compliance; LVEDWT = left ventricular end-diastolic wall thickness.
Reproduced with permission from Reference 14.

ter body surface area is not clearly outside a normal range,[9] the absolute volume, and increased LV posterior wall thickness reflect a significant increase in LV mass, presumably secondary to hypertrophy. LV end-diastolic circumferential wall stress is modestly elevated.[10] LV end-diastolic chamber compliance is well below the normal lower limit of 2.8 compliance units.[11]

Thus, in one setting pulmonary and systemic vascular congestion develop as a consequence of chronic circulatory volume overload in association with LV hypertrophy, diminished chamber compliance, and preserved systolic function. Chest roentgenograms of such a patient are shown in Figure 2, which illustrates the changes in heart size and pulmonary vascularity with weight cycling over a period of 8 years. The degree of volume overload paralleled the change in body weight. In another setting, chronic volume overload, sometimes with pressure overload as well, and long-term increase in LV wall stress may result in LV systolic dysfunction, as well as diastolic and CHF in the usual sense.[7] Prognosis would seem less favorable in the latter group, but this is not well documented.

The natural history of this condition is characterized by repeated bouts of pulmonary and systemic congestive symptoms, usually responding to transient weight reduction over a period of at least several years or more.[12] With recurrent bouts of congestion, atrial fibrillation[13–15] or flutter[16] tend to develop. A hypoventilation syndrome may precede or follow the onset of circulatory congestive state in extremely obese subjects with an incidence of about 10% in cross-sectional study.[6]

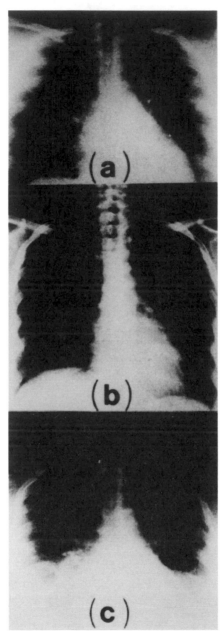

Figure 2. Serial chest x-ray films of a 29-year-old woman (weight 184 kg) who initially presented with severe congestive symptoms, cardiomegaly, and pulmonary edema **(panel a)**. Two years later, at a weight of 157 kg, she experienced marked

Chronic hypoxemia and hypercapnia, as a consequence of hypoventilation in these subjects, result in superimposition of pulmonary vasoconstriction upon the pre-existing hemodynamic alterations secondary to LV dysfunction, thus, exacerbating pulmonary hypertension. While isolated cor pulmonale does not occur in those subjects,[1] occasionally the predominant involvement may be right-sided, which predispositions to biventricular hypertrophy. As the condition progresses, somnolence is present to an increasing degree and may become incapacitating.[6, 12] Although carbon dioxide retention may play a role in the pathogenesis of somnolence, there is no clear relation to carbon dioxide arterial tension levels and severe somnolence may develop with normal levels.[6] Mental confusion and disorientation are frequent, at least in part related to cerebral edema. Coma may supervene in the preterminal phase.[12]

On physical examination, cyanosis and Cheyne-Stokes respiration are common. Conjunctional suffusion, retinal venous congestion, and papilledema may be present.[17, 18] Elevation of jugular venous pressure, although present, may be difficult to appraise. Crepitant pulmonary rales are common. Presystolic (S_4) or summation gallop rhythm may be present on cardiac examination, but murmurs are infrequent. Hepatomegaly, ascites, and brawny leg edema are routinely observed. Since neither the history nor findings on examination serve to differentiate those with combined systolic and diastolic LV function from those with predominantly diastolic dysfunction, appraisal of ventricular function by echocardiography or other noninterventional means is useful from both diagnostic and therapeutic standpoints.

The absence of evidence for LV hypertrophy in the electrocardiogram (ECG) of the morbidly obese subject is a striking feature, especially since its degree may be massive (Figure 3). Comparing ECG criteria for LV hypertrophy with echocardiographic measurements of LV wall thickness, mass, and dimension, the presence of one or more criteria is highly specific for LV hypertrophy, but sensitivity is extremely low.[19] Similar findings apply to the right ventricle. There may be a ten-

---

improvement in symptoms. With a decrease in heart size and regression of pulmonary congestion (**panel b**). However, cardiomegaly and pulmonary congestion recurred with weight gain 6 years later (**panel c**). An echocardiogram recorded at age 43 years and 195 kg weight showed an LV diastolic dimension of 4.8 cm, with an increase in wall thickness to 1.5 cm and a reduction in E to F slope to 30 mm/s, which suggests lowered LV chamber compliance. However, indices of LV contractile state were in a normal range: ejection fraction 64% and velocity of circumferential fiber shortening 1.36 circumferences/s. By age 48, she had developed atrial fibrillation. (Reproduced from Reference 14 with permission.)

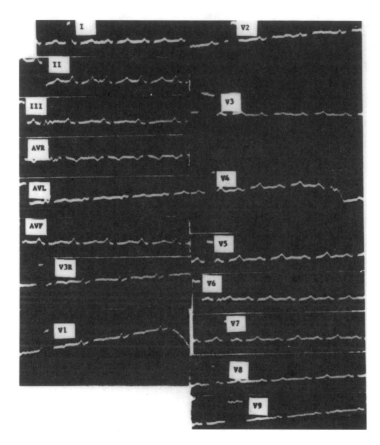

Figure 3. Electrocardiogram of a man (weight 183 kg) presenting congestive heart failure. Rhythm is sinus and QRS axis is approximately 90° in the frontal plane. There is no ECG evidence to suggest the severe degree of LV hypertrophy (heart weight 1100 g, LV wall thickness 25 mm) found at necropsy. (Reproduced from Reference 14 with permission.)

dency to leftward shift in the P, QRS, and T axes,[20, 21] or a normal axis.[18] Voltage in the ECG may be minimally lower with slight diminution in the amplitude of the spatial QRS vector,[20, 21] but the vectorcardiographic features may not differ from the normal.[22] Flattening of the T waves in the inferolateral leads,[21] and left atrial abnormality (terminal forces of P wave ≥ −0.04 mm/sec) may be present.[23] In some patients with obesity hypoventilation, axis deviation to the right is observed.[18] With significant weight reduction (30 to 40 kg), QRS and P wave amplitudes may fall[21, 22] and T waves in the inferolateral leads may normalize.[21] Thus, the most notable aspects of the ECG in morbid obesity are the modest deviations from normal and its failure to reflect the dramatic changes in cardiac anatomy that take place. This has been ascribed to the effect of the anatomy of the thorax (increased fat tissue mass) upon the transmission of electrical impulses.

Chest roentgenograms of morbidly obese subjects frequently demonstrate cardiomegaly (Figure 2).[6] Comparison of the observed transverse cardiac diameters with normal values from the Ungerleider-Clark table,[24] taking height and predicted ideal weight of the obese subject, regularly shows greater diameter in the obese subject (Figure 4). Two-thirds of the patient diameters shown in Figure 4 are 20% to 40% greater than predicted at ideal weight, with an overall range of 10% to 55% increase. There is a quasilinear relation between cardiac diameter and body weight, with an increment of 1 mm in cardiac diameter per 3 lbs in weight.

Excess adipose tissue of the thorax and upper abdomen, as well as displacement of the heart to a more transverse position by elevation of the diaphragm, make for limitation in echocardiographic assessment of cardiac morphology and function in extremely obese subjects. In one study of markedly obese persons, using a dedicated M-mode echocardiograph and 2.25 MHz transducer, both LV septum and posterior wall were visualized in only 36% of cases, and neither septum nor posterior wall in 42%.[25] Use of two-dimensional echocardiography and concurrent

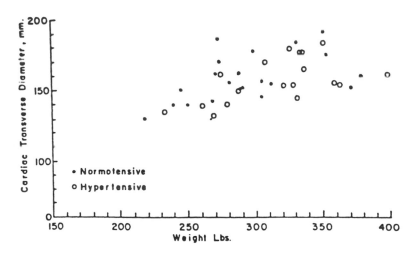

Figure 4. Relation between the roentgeographic estimate of cardiac transverse diameter and body weight in forth extremely obese subjects. (Reproduced from Reference 6 with permission.)

M-mode enhances the frequency of anatomic visualization.[26] Table 2 demonstrates feasibility data of concurrent two-dimensional/M-mode echocardiography in 82 morbidly obese patients. A complete examination was attainable in 70% of patients and key cardiac structures could be imaged in 80% to 98% of cases. Ability to record a full circumference of endocardial echoes in one or more views was possible in half of all patients studied. Recording from the third or fourth intercostal space at the right sternal border was necessary for parasternal images in one-third, and at the anterior or midaxillary line in three-fourths for the apical view. Currently, there are no feasibility studies for Doppler, color-flow Doppler, or transesophageal imaging in extremely obese subjects.

The mode of exitus in morbidly obese subjects has been addressed in several autopsy studies. Death due to CHF in nine "extremely" obese subjects, without other apparent cause, was first reported by Smith and Willius in 1933.[27] In a subsequent autopsy report of 12 morbidly obese subjects, 3 died of CHF.[28] A retrospective survey of 3514 consecutive autopsies at a Veterans Administration Hospital reported 9 patients weighing 300 lbs or more. Severe pulmonary and systemic congestion were present in all but 1, and evidences of CHF had been present in 6 antemortem.[12]

There are several case reports documenting sudden death in morbidly obese patients with cardiomegaly and pulmonary congestion at necropsy[13,15,29-31] with no apparent precipitating cause. However, the frequency of sudden death in this setting was first observed by MacGregor and colleagues[18] who reported five such cases in a group of 22 morbidly obese subjects. Subsequently, a study of 12 patients weighing 300 lbs or more at autopsy also documented sudden death in 5 with cardiomegaly and pulmonary congestion, but did not indicate apparent precipitating cause of death.[32] A survey of morbidly obese persons undergoing surgery to achieve weight loss reports 60 sudden deaths among 50,134 patients.[33] The calculated annual mortality rate for this group was 40 times higher than that estimated for a matched nonobese population. Although 22 of these deaths occurred in the first 10 days postoperatively, 8 occurred preoperatively and late deaths were recorded up to 22 months postoperatively. In 36 instances, autopsy demonstrated increased heart weights with increased LV wall thickness in 9 of 14 patients, in which wall thickness was recorded. A precipitating cause was not found in any case. Whenever terminal events were monitored, cardiac arrests were secondary to ventricular tachycardia or fibrillation. Torsade de pointes was present in three electrocardiographic tracings. An adjusted QT interval (QTc) was longer than 0.430 seconds (upper normal 0.425 seconds) in 29 of 38 tracings, which

Table 2
Feasibility of Concurrent Two-dimensional/M-mode
Echocardiography in 82 Extremely-obese Patients

	Frequency of Visualization(%)	
Cardiac Structure	M-Mode Echocardiography	Two-Dimensional Echocardiography
Interventricular septum alone	84	93
Left ventricular posterior wall alone	83	88
Interventricular septum and left ventricular posterior wall	80	83
Right ventricular anterior wall	82	85
Measurable left ventricular internal dimension		
Diastole	80	83
Systole	80	80
Both	80	80
Measurable left atrial dimension	98	98
Measurable right ventricular internal dimension	78	83
Measurable right atrial dimension	—	79
Aortic Valve		
Left coronary cusp alone	—	—
Noncoronary cusp alone	7	—
Right coronary cusp alone	4	—
Right and noncoronary cusps	83	—
All three cusps	—	90
Mitral Valve		
Anterior leaflet alone	10	7
Posterior leaflet alone	0	0
Both leaflets	83	93
Pulmonic Valve		
Posterior cusp alone	65	67
Anterior cusp alone	0	0
Both cusps	67	0
Tricuspid Valve		
Anterior leaflet alone	51	0
Septal leaflet alone	—	0
Posterior leaflet alone	0	0
Anterior and posterior leaflets	10	12
Anterior and septal leaflets	—	85
All three leaflets	—	17
Pericardium		
Anterior	83	—
Posterior	88	—
Anterior and posterior	80	—

possibly predisposed to arrhythmia. In a retrospective survey of sudden death cases in obese subjects at the Armed Forces Institute of Pathology, the commonest findings were eccentric LV hypertrophy and myocyte hypertrophy.[34] Two postmortem studies of the cardiac construction system in morbidly obese subjects[15,35] demonstrated similar findings: fatty infiltration of the approaches to the sinus node with collections of mononuclear cells, with fatty changes and fibrosis in relation to the atrioventricular mode and bifurcation of the bundle branch. In one case it was postulated that fatty infiltration involved the sinus node and atrial conduction bundles had led to atrial fibrillation,[15] as fat infiltration of the myocardium may be associated with conduction defect.[36,37] There is evidence to suggest that myocardial hypertrophy may be associated with an increased incidence of sudden death.[40] Since ventricular fibrillation is frequently preceded by ventricular tachycardia, increased ventricular ectopy in obese hypertensives with hypertrophy, versus without, has been suggested as a means of identifying those at increased risk and fence candidates for more aggressive treatment.[39] However, it has not been demonstrated that suppression of ventricular ectopy with antiarrhythmic therapy or control of risk factors prevents sudden cardiac death.

Summary and Conclusions

Morbid obesity appears to be associated with the development of a circulatory congestive state in approximately 10% of cases in cross-sectional study. However, postmortem findings suggest that the incidence is higher on long-term follow-up. This congestive state is characterized by marked eccentric LV, and sometimes right ventricular, hypertrophy. LV diastolic dysfunction is present in all cases, while systolic dysfunction is present in some cases. Exacerbation or amelioration of congestive symptoms and signs are precipitated by weight gain or loss, respectively, with cycles in some cases over many years. In about 10% of morbidly obese subjects a hypoventilation syndrome develops, which superimposes increased pulmonary vascular resistance secondary to hypoxemia and respiratory acidosis upon the preexisting hemodynamic alterations due to LV dysfunction. Electrocardiographic studies of morbidly obese subjects have demonstrated no change or modest diminution in amplitude of the spatial QRS vector, flattening of T waves in the inferolateral leads, and left atrial abnormality. Left- or right-axis deviation may be present. The most notable feature is failure of the ECG to reflect the dramatic changes in left or right ventricular hypertrophy present anatomically. Increase in cardiac diameter or chest roentgenogram as compared with that for ideal weight is regularly present, with a quasilinear relation between increment in diameter and body weight. A complete transthoracic echocardiographic examination is attainable in 70% of patients and key cardiac structures can be visualized in 80% to 98% of severely obese individuals.

Although death may come about in association with progression of heart failure, there is a predisposition to sudden death with or without a congestive circulatory state. In monitored instances, this has been due to ventricular tachycardia or fibrillation. In the absence of other identifiable factors, the mechanism of sudden death has been linked to myocardial hypertrophy or to fatty infiltration of myocardium and conduction system. While hypertrophied myocardium may serve as an arrhythmogenic substrate for ventricular ectopy, it is not known whether this holds for areas in which fatty infiltration has involved myocardium or the conduction system. Elucidation of the mechanism of sudden death requires further study.

References

1. Alexander JK. Obesity and the heart. *Curr Prob Cardiol* 5:1–41, 1980.
2. Kaltman AJ, Goldring RM: Role of circulatory congestion in the cardiorespiratory failure of obesity. *Am J Med* 60:645–653, 1976.
3. Rochester DF, Enson Y: Current concepts in the pathogenosis of the obesity-hypoventilation syndrome. *Am J Med* 57:402–420, 1974.
4. White RE, Alexander JK: Body oxygen consumption and pulmonary ventilation in obese subjects. *J Appl Physiol* 20:197–201, 1965.
5. Turell DJ, Austin RC, Alexander JK: Cardiorespiratory response of very obese subjects to treadmill exercise. *J Lab Clin Med* 64:107–113, 1964.
6. Alexander JK, Amad KH, Cole VW: Observations on some clinical features of extreme obesity, with particular reference to cardiorespiratory effects. *Am J Med* 32:512–524, 1962.
7. Alexander JK, Woodard CB, Quinones MA, et al: Heart failure from obesity. In Mancini M, Lewis B, Cartaldo F (eds): *Medical Complications of Obesity.* Academic Press, London, 1978, pp. 179–187.
8. Ford LE: Heart size. *Circ Res* 39:297–303, 1976.
9. Dodge HT, Baxley WA: Left ventricular volume and mass and their significance in heart disease. *Am J Cardiol* 23:528–537, 1969.
10. Grossman W, Jones D, McLaurin LP: Wall stress and patterns of hypertrophy in the human left ventricle. *J Clin Invest* 56:56–64, 1974.
11. Gaash WH, Quinones MA, Waisser E, et al: Diastolic compliance of the left ventricle in man. *Am J Cardiol* 36:193–201, 1975.

12. Alexander JK, Pettigrove JK: Obesity and congestive heart failure. *Geriatrics* 22:101–108, 1967.
13. Carroll D: A peculiar type of cardiopulmonary failure associated with obesity. *Am J Med* 21:819–824, 1956.
14. Alexander JK: The cardiomyopathy of obesity. *Prog Cardiovasc Dis* 27: 325–334, 1985.
15. James TN, Frame B, Coates EO: De subitaneis Mortibus III. Pickwickian syndrome. *Circulation* 48:1311–1320, 1973.
16. Estes EH Jr., Sickes HO, McIntosh HD, et al: Reversible cardiopulmonary syndrome with extreme obesity. *Circulation* 16:179–187, 1957.
17. Meyer JA, Gotham J, Tazaki Y, et al: Cardiorespiratory syndrome of extreme obesity with papilledema. *Neurology* 11:950–958, 1961.
18. MacGregor MI, Block AJ, Ball WC: Serious complications and death in the Pickwickian syndrome. *John Hopkins Med J* 126:279–295, 1970.
19. Nath A, Alpert MA, Terry BE, et al: Sensitivity and specificity of electrocardiographic criteria for left and right ventricular hypertrophy in morbid obesity. *Am J Cardiol* 62:126–130, 1988.
20. Axelrod MA, Alexander JK: The electrocardiogram and cardiac anatomy in obesity. *Clin Res* 13:25, 1965.
21. Eisenstein I, Edelstein J, Sarma R, et al: The electrocardiogram in obesity. *J Electrocardiol* 15:115–118, 1982.
22. Brohet CR, Tuna N: Quantitative analysis of the vectorcardiogram in obesity. The effects of weight reduction. *J Electrocardiol* 8:1–11, 1975.
23. Lavie CJ, Amodea C, Ventura HO, et al: Left atrial abnormalities indicating diastolic ventricular dysfunction in cardiomyopathy of obesity. *Chest* 92:1042–1046, 1987.
24. Ungerleider HE, Clark PC: A study of the transverse diameter of the heart silhouette with prediction based on the teleoroentgenogram. *Am Heart J* 17:92–98, 1939.
25. Zema MJ, Caccavano M: Feasibility of M-mode echocardiographic examination in markedly obese adults: Prospective study of 50 patients. *J Clin Ultrasound* 10:31–36, 1982.
26. Alpert MA, Kelly DL: Value and limitations of echocardiography in the assessment of obese patients. *Echocardiography* 3:261–272, 1986.
27. Smith HL, Willius FA: Adiposity of the heart. *Arch Intern Med* 52:911–931, 1933.
28. Amad KH, Brennan JC, Alexander JK: The cardiac pathology of chronic exogenous obesity. *Circulation* 32:740–745, 1965.
29. Counihan TB: Heart failure due to extreme obesity. *Br Heart J* 18:425–426, 1956.
30. Jenab M, Lade RI, Chiga M, et al: Cardiorespiratory syndrome of obesity in a child. *Pediatrics* 24:23–30, 1959.
31. Huang TY: Cardiac pathology in the sudden death of an extremely obese person. *Indiana Med J* 14:860–865, 1986.
32. Warnes CH, Roberts WC: The heart in massive (more than 300 pounds or 136 kilograms) obesity: Analysis of 12 patients studied at necropsy. *Am J Cardiol* 54:1087–1091, 1984.
33. Drenick EJ, Fisher JS: Sudden cardiac arrest in morbidly obese surgical patients unexplained after autopsy. *Am J Surg* 155:720–726, 1988.

34. Duflou J, Virmani R, Rabin I, et al: Sudden death as a result of heart disease in morbid obesity. *Am Heart J* 130:306–313, 1995.
35. Bharati S, Lev M: Cardiac conduction system involvement in sudden death of obese young people. *Am Heart J* 129(2):273–281, 1995.
36. Spain DM, Catheast RT: Heart block caused by fat infiltration of the interventricular septum "cor adiposum". *Am Heart J* 32:659–664, 1946.
37. Balsaver AM, Morales AR, Whitehouse FW: Fat infiltration of myocardium as a cause of cardiac conduction defect. *Am J Cardiol* 19:261–265, 1967.
38. Anderson KP: Sudden death, hypertension, and hypertrophy. *J Cardiovasc Pharmacol* 6(Suppl 3):S498–S503, 1984.
39. Messerli F, Nunez B, Ventura H, et al: Overweight and sudden death. Increased ventricular ectopy in cardiomyopathy of obesity. *Arch Intern Med* 147:1725–1728, 1987.
40. Oliver MF: Lack of impact of prevention on sudden death. *J Am Coll Cardiol* 5:150B–154B, 1985.

Chapter 10

Obesity and
Sleep-disordered Breathing

Steven M. Koenig, M.D.
Paul M. Suratt, M.D.

The classic example of a disorder due to abnormal breathing during sleep is the obstructive sleep apnea (OSA) syndrome. The OSA syndrome is characterized by repetitive episodes of complete or partial upper airway obstruction during sleep, which results in significant physiological consequences such as sleep fragmentation and oxyhemoglobin desaturation. Once thought to be an uncommon disorder, a recent community-based study estimated that 2% to 4% of randomly chosen middle-aged adults have this condition.[1] In addition, evidence indicates that this disorder is associated with increased mortality as well as cardiovascular morbidity.[2-5]

Although numerous factors and conditions may predispose to OSA syndrome, excess body fat is by far the most common. If defined as a body mass index (BMI) greater than 28 kg/m^2, obesity is present in 60% to 90% of OSA patients evaluated in sleep clinics.[6-9] In one study, obesity was a better predictor of severity of sleep apnea than both gender and age.[9] In another investigation, an increase in BMI of one standard deviation was associated with a fourfold increase in risk of OSA.[1] Finally, numerous studies have indicated that OSA generally improves with weight loss.[10-16]

Approximately 10% of patients with OSA develop chronic daytime hypoventilation, defined as a sustained increase in arterial carbon dioxide tension (PaCO$_2$) exceeding 45 mm Hg.[17] Those that do are typically morbidly obese. The term obesity-hypoventilation sydrome (OHS) is used to describe this combination of obesity and hypoventilation. Al-

From: Alpert MA, and Alexander JK, (eds). *The Heart and Lung in Obesity*. Armonk, NY: Futura Publishing Company, Inc., © 1998.

though the majority of individuals with OHS have concomitant OSA syndrome, OSA is not an essential feature of OHS.[18]

The purpose of this chapter is to outline the underlying pathophysiology, presenting symptoms and signs, diagnosis and treatment of OSA syndrome and OHS, with emphasis on the role and importance of obesity in these conditions. Because sleep-disordered breathing is clearly a major public health problem, and because many cases are often unsuspected, it is essential that physicians as well as the public at large become more aware of the clinical presentation of these very common disorders.

Definitions

An apnea is defined as the complete or near-complete cessation of airflow that lasts for at least 10 seconds.[19] Although there is no consensus for its exact definition, a hypopnea is reasonably defined as a decrease in airflow of 30% to 50% from baseline, lasting at least 10 seconds.[19–21] These abnormal respiratory events may or may not be accompanied by oxyhemoglobin desaturation of 3% to 4% or more. Although apneas may be associated with greater oxyhemoglobin desaturation, hypopneas are associated with the similar sequelae and are treated in the same manner (Figures 1A and 1B).

Apneas and hypopneas are further divided into obstructive, central and mixed.[19,22] They are considered obstructive if there is continued or increasing respiratory effort despite absent or diminished airflow, central, if there is absent respiratory effort (Figure 2). An event is labeled mixed if it begins as a central apnea or hypopnea and is terminated by an obstructive event.

The upper airway resistance syndrome (UARS) is a newly described syndrome in which patients have repetitive episodes of narrowing of the upper airway that causes arousals from sleep that in turn lead to excessive daytime sleepiness or tiredness.[23] Although people with this condition do not have apneas or hypopneas, the narrowing of their airway causes the respiratory muscles to increase their work to the point where an arousal occurs. At the present time, this condition can be reliably diagnosed only by measuring esophageal pressure. In this syndrome, esophageal pressure becomes more negative with each inspiration, indicating increased respiratory effort, until an arousal from sleep occurs (Figure 1C).

The term hypoventilation is utilized when oxyhemoglobin desatura-

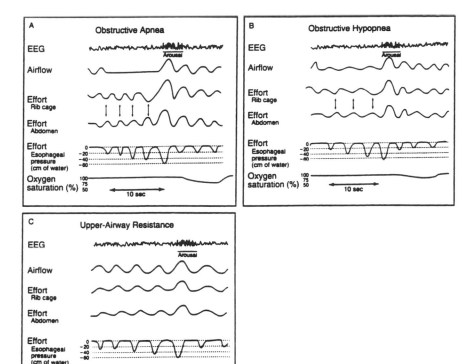

Figure 1. Manifestations of upper-airway closure. **Panel A** depicts obstructive apnea. Increasing ventilatory effort is seen in the rib cage, the abdomen, and the level of esophageal pressure (measured with an esophageal balloon), despite lack of oronasal airflow. Arousal on the electroencephalogram (EEG) is associated with increasing ventilatory effort, as indicated by the esophageal pressure. Oxyhemoglobin desaturation follows the termination of apnea. Note that during apnea, the movements of the rib cage and the abdomen (Effort) are in opposite directions (**arrows**) as a result of attempts to breath against a closed airway. Once the airway opens in response to arousal, rib cage and abdominal movements become synchronous. **Panel B** depicts obstructive hypopnea. Decreased airflow is associated with increasing ventilatory effort (reflected by the esophageal pressure) and subsequent arousal on the EEG. Rib cage and abdominal movements are in opposite directions during hypopnea (arrows), reflecting increasingly difficult breathing against a partially closed airway. Rib cage and abdominal movements become synchronous after arousal produces airway opening. Oxyhemoglobin desaturation follows the termination of hypopnea. **Panel C** depicts upper-airway resistance. Asynchronous movements of the rib cage and abdomen and a substantial decrease in airflow are not seen. Arousal on the EEG is associated with increasing ventilatory effort due to increased airway resistance, as reflected by the esophageal pressure. There is no significant oxyhemoglobin desaturation. (Fom Strollo PJ Jr et al. *N Engl J Med* 4:99–104, 1996, with permission.)

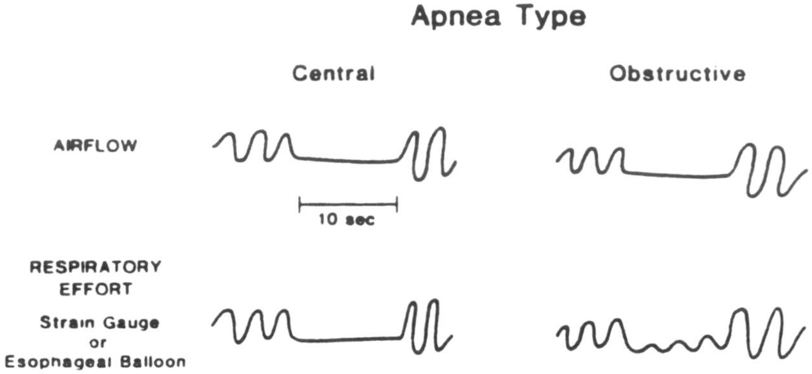

Apnea Type

Central   Obstructive

Figure 2. The relation between airflow and respiratory effort in both central and obstructive apnea. During a central apnea there is cessation of airflow for at least 10 seconds with no associated ventilatory effort. An obstructive apnea is defined as a similar cessation of airflow, but with continued respiratory effort. (From White DP. *Clin Chest Med* 6:624, 1985, with permission.)

tion (and elevated arterial carbon dioxide tension, if measured) is present, but there are no abnormalities in the pattern of breathing. That is, there is a relatively constant or slowly diminishing oxyhemoglobin desaturation, without the cyclic, episodic or repetitive changes in oxygen saturation associated with apneas and hypopneas or the arousal that terminates these abnormal breathing events (Figure 3). Because everyone hypoventilates somewhat when they fall asleep, and often with rapid eye movements during rapid eye movement (REM)-sleep, hypoventilation is considered abnormal only if associated with clinically significant oxyhemoglobin desaturation (i.e. less than 88% to 90%) or hypercapnia.

Snoring is an inspiratory sound produced by vibration of the soft portions of the oro and nasopharynx. For snoring to occur, both the proper structure, for example, a long floppy uvula and soft palate, as well as exposure to an inspiratory pressure negative enough to set these tissues in motion must be present. The reason more than 80% of individuals with OSA snore is that the most common site of upper airway abnormality and narrowing is the region around the soft palate.

Indicators of the severity of sleep-disordered breathing include the apnea index, which is the number of apneas per hour of sleep, the hypopnea index, which is the number of hypopneas per hour of sleep, the respiratory disturbance index (RDI), which is the number of apneas plus hypopneas per hour of sleep and the oxyhemoglobin desaturation

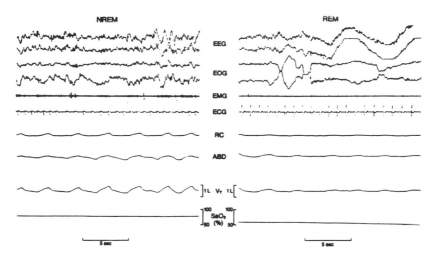

Figure 3. Polysomnographic recording from a postpolio patient demonstrating hypoventilation. The channels show (from top to bottom) electroencephalogram (EEG), electro-oculogram (EOG), submental electromyogram (EMG), electrocardiogram (ECG), excursion of the rib cage (RC), abdomen (ABD) and their sum (VT), and arterial oxyhemoglobin saturation (SaO_2). The pattern of breathing is rapid and shallow, and during REM sleep the baseline saturation falls but remains steady. This is accompanied by decreased excursion of both the rib cage and abdomen. (From Goldstein RS, et al. *Am Rev Respir Dis* 135:1049–1055, 1987, with permission.)

index, which is the number of oxyhemoglobin desaturation episodes 3% or 4% or less per hour. Patient's with the Pickwickian syndrome first described by Burwell in 1956, complain of daytime hypersomnolence and dyspnea; are morbidly obese, plethoric (from polycythemia) and cyanotic (from hypoxemia); have both hypoxemia and hypercapnia on arterial blood gases; and have signs of pulmonary hypertension and right ventricular failure.[24] The term "Pickwickian" is best reserved for those individuals on the severe end of the OHS spectrum.

The multiple sleep latency test (MSLT) is used in the assessment and diagnosis of disorders of excessive sleepiness. A series of four or five opportunities to sleep is administered to a patient at 2-hour intervals using standard procedures. Sleepiness is measured as the speed of falling asleep (sleep latency); the presence of REM sleep is also noted. A mean sleep latency for all naps of less than 5 minutes is considered severely sleepy; 5 to 8 minutes moderately sleepy; 8 to 10 minutes mildly sleepy; and greater than 10 minutes normal. The appearance of REM sleep in two or more naps is suggestive of narcolepsy.[25]

Pathogenesis

Obstructive Sleep Apnea

Narrowing of the human pharynx or upper airway is responsible for all the consequences associated with OSA.[27] The pharynx is typically divided into three segments: the nasopharynx (end of the nasal septum to the margin of the soft palate); the oropharynx (free margin of the soft palate to the tip of the epiglottis), which is divided into the retropalatal and retroglossal regions; and the hypopharynx (tip of the epiglottis to the vocal cords) (Figure 4). In one study, 75% of patients had more than one site of narrowing, the retropalatal region or velopharynx being the most common site.[26]

Because narrowing of the human pharynx is the underlying cause of OSA, individuals with this condition must have some abnormality or abnormalities of the determinants of the caliber of their upper airway. According to the "Balance of Pressures" concept proposed by Remmers et al., and Brouillette and Thach, there are five major determinants of the caliber of the upper airway (Figure 5): (1) the baseline pharyngeal area, which is determined by both craniofacial and soft tissue struc-

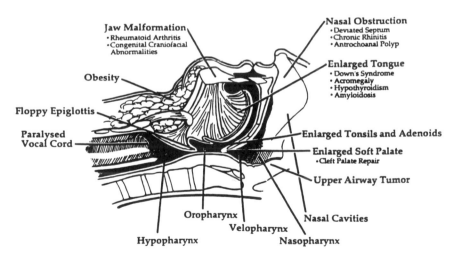

Figure 4. Diagram of the upper airway, which shows the different segments of the pharynx and indicates the variety of upper airway abnormalities reported to cause obstructive sleep apnea. (From Fleetham JA. *Clin Chest Med* 13:400, 1992, with permission.)

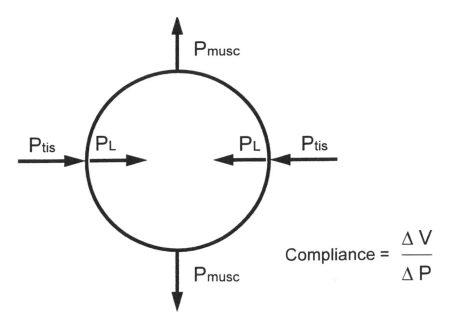

Figure 5. Determinants of upper airway caliber. PL = intraluminal pressure; Ptis = pressure in the tissues surrounding the pharyngeal wall; Pmusc = pressure exerted by the pharyngeal dilating muscles; D V = change in volume; D P = change in pressure.

tures (Figure 4); (2) the compliance or collapsibility of the airway; (3) the luminal pressure (PL), which on inspiration is negative, due to the upwardly transmitted negative intrapleural pressure, and tends to narrow the airway; (4) the pressure in the tissues surrounding the pharyngeal wall (Ptis), which can be positive, and also tends to collapse the airway; examples include compression of the upper airway by the lateral pharyngeal fat pad, a large neck, the effect of gravity on submandibular fat, and a large tongue confined to a small oral cavity; and (5) the pressure exerted by the pharyngeal dilating muscles (Pmusc), which is directed outwards, and functions to increase cross sectional area and decrease pharyngeal compliance.[26–28] In addition, there is *theoretical* evidence that the *shape* of the upper airway is also important. Compared with the elliptically shaped airways of normal controls, the long axis of which is oriented transversely, the pharynx of patients with OSA has more of an anteroposterior or longitudinal alignment. Such an orientation could decrease Pmusc by diminishing the mechanical effectiveness of upper airway muscle contraction.[29,30] Finally, lung volume independently influences upper airway caliber, resistance and compliance. Decreased lung volume decreases tracheal tug (caudal traction) on pharyngeal soft tissue structures. This in turn leads to a decrease in the area of the pharynx, an increase in upper airway resistance,[31] and an increase in pharyngeal compliance or collapsibility.[31–34]

Although narrowing of the human upper airway is the primary event in OSA, the occurrence of oxyhemoglobin desaturation during the abnormal respiratory event is dependent on several other factors. The primary determinants of oxyhemoglobin desaturation with hypoventilation, an apnea or hypopnea include: (1) the length of the abnormal respiratory event, the longer the event, the more likely oxygen desaturation will occur; (2) the type of respiratory event, obstructive events being associated with respiratory effort and therefore greater oxygen consumption than central events; (3) the quantity of oxygen stored in the lungs, which is proportional to the lung volume and the fractional concentration of oxygen in the alveoli (a small lung volume is associated with greater desaturation than a large lung volume); (4) the mixed venous oxygen saturation, the lower this saturation, the more rapid the rate of fall in arterial oxyhemoglobin desaturation; and (5) the baseline arterial oxygen saturation; the lower the value, the closer you are to the knee of the oxyhemoglobin dissociation curve at the start of the abnormal respiratory event, and the more likely you are to desaturate (Figure 6).[35]

Although numerous changes occur during sleep, those most important in the pathogenesis of OSA are the decrease in both Pmusc and lung volume associated with sleep onset.[36–38] The latter exacerbates the decreased lung volume associated with assumption of the supine position. In addition, the effect of gravity on a large neck or parapharyngeal fat may increase Ptis. The overall result is an increase in upper airway resistance due to the decrease in cross-sectional area and increase in compliance or collapsibility of the upper airway.[38,39] Stiffer, smaller lungs and resultant atelectasis may also cause a decrease in baseline oxyhemoglobin saturation and the other determinants of the degree of oxygen desaturation with an apnea, hypopnea, or hypoventilation.

The pharynx of persons without OSA has sufficient "reserve" to tolerate this increase in upper airway resistance and collapsibility associated with sleep. In contrast, individuals with OSA have some predisposing condition, either a pharynx with a baseline area that is too small, or an abnormality in one or more of the determinants of upper airway caliber mentioned above. Thus, when they fall asleep, their upper airway cannot tolerate this decrease in Pmusc, lung volume and increase in Ptis. The result is an upper airway resistance of sufficient magnitude to cause physiological consequences (see below).

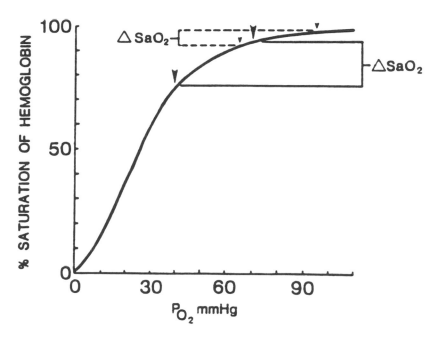

Figure 6. Affect of initial PO_2 on amount of arterial oxygen desaturation seen. Because of the shape of the oxygen-hemoglobin dissociation curve, the amount of decrease in SaO_2 seen with equivalent decrease in PO_2 is different for different starting PO_2's. When the starting PO_2 is near or below the "elbow" of the curve more desaturation is seen. (Reproduced from Reference 35 with permission.

Those factors that have been shown to predispose to OSA and how they interact with the determinants of upper airway caliber described above are listed in Table 1. See also Figure 4, for examples of upper airway anatomic abnormalities that can predispose to OSA.

Since REM sleep is associated with greater muscle hypotonia compared with non-REM sleep, apneas and hypopneas are more likely to occur in REM.[40] The more impaired ventilatory responses to hypoxia and hypercapnia that occur in REM also contribute to the longer duration of abnormal respiratory events and the presence of post apneic hypoventilation in REM.[41,42] The result is more frequent and more severe episodes of increased upper airway resistance and oxyhemoglobin desaturation compared with non-REM sleep.

To predispose to OSA, obesity must influence one or more of the above mentioned determinants of upper airway caliber, or of the degree of oxyhemoglobin desaturation associated with a given abnormal res-

Table 1
Factors Predisposing to Obstructive Sleep Apnea
Syndrome and How They Interact with the
Determinants of Pharyngeal Caliber

Predisposing Factor	Awake Pharyngeal Area	Luminal Pressure (PL)	Tissue Pressure (Ptis)	Pharyngeal Muscle Dilating Force (Pmusc)	Pharyngeal Compliance
Obesity	Decreased	—	Increased	Decreased ?	Increased
Neuro-muscular Disease	Decreased	—	—	Decreased	Increased
Alcohol	Decreased	—	—	Decreased	—
Sedative-hypnotics	—	—	—	Decreased	—
Nasal Congestion	—	Increased	—	—	—
Abnormal Anatomy	Decreased	—	—	—	—
Supine Position	Decreased	—	Increased	—	—
Sleep Deprivation	—	—	—	Decreased	Increased
Hypothyroidism	Decreased	—	Increased	Decreased	—
Acromegaly	Decreased	—	Increased	—	—

piratory event. As it turns out, there is evidence that obesity can influence all of these determinants, which explains not only why obesity is the most common factor predisposing to OSA, but why obese individuals with OSA are more likely to have more severe clinical consequences than their non-obese counterparts (Figure 7).

Although it is unclear whether the predominant mechanism is increased Ptis or simply excessive parapharyngeal tissue without an increase in Ptis, the majority of studies indicate that compared to weight-matched controls, obese patients with OSA have a smaller baseline pharyngeal cross sectional area. This narrowing is located predominantly in the retropalatal region.[28,43] Logic would dictate that excessive adipose tissue should be the cause of this decreased area, and there is evidence to support this hypothesis. Using magnetic resonance imaging (MRI), which can distinguish soft tissue from fat, one study indicated that compared with weight-matched controls, obese patients with OSA had excess fat deposition in the soft palate, tongue, and in areas

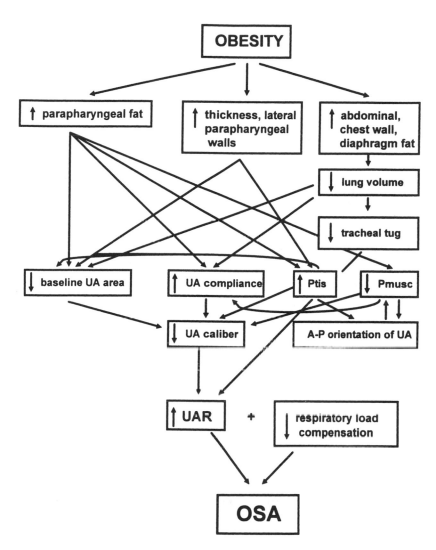

Figure 7. The pathophysiological role of obesity in the obstructive sleep apnea syndrome. UA = upper airway; UAR = upper airway resistance; OSA = obstructive sleep apnea; Ptis = pressure in tissues surrounding the pharyngeal wall; Pmusc = pressure exerted by pharyngeal dilating muscles.

posterior and lateral to the oropharynx at the level of the palate.[44] Two other MRI studies confirmed the smaller baseline pharyngeal area in obese subjects with OSA, and also demonstrated the presence of a larger volume of adipose tissue adjacent to the pharyngeal airway.[45,46] Moreover, not only did the volume of this parapharyngeal fat correlate with the degree of OSA, but weight loss resulted in a substantial decrease in both pharyngeal adipose tissue volume and severity of OSA.[46] In addition, surgical specimens from individuals with OSA who underwent uvulopalatopharyngoplasty (UPPP) (see below) have demonstrated increased fat in the soft palate.[47]

In contrast, although Schwab et al.[48] confirmed that airway size is smaller in patients with sleep apnea, their findings indicated that it was the thickness of the lateral Ptis and not the size of the soft palate, tongue or parapharyngeal fat pads that was the major anatomic factor causing airway narrowing in apneics. Moreover, using a proton spectroscopic technique called HUPSPEC with MRI, they demonstrated that this increased thickness of the lateral Ptis was not secondary to increased fat infiltration or edema.[49,50] He went on to hypothesize that obesity may predispose to sleep apnea by increasing the size of the upper airway soft tissue structures themselves, rather than by the direct deposition of fat in the parapharyngeal fat pads or by fat pads compressing the lateral walls of the pharynx. Thus, although most evidence supports a smaller baseline upper airway caliber in obese patients, the exact mechanism of this narrowing remains to be defined.

Fat might also encroach on the upper airway lumen and alter its shape without necessarily reducing its diameter. With MRI, differences in pharyngeal shape but not in cross-sectional area have been documented between obese patients and normal weight controls.[30] When the pharynx was viewed in coronal section, the airways of normal awake controls were in the shape of an ellipse, with its long axis oriented transversely. In contrast, awake OSA patients had elliptically shaped airways oriented in an anteroposterior or longitudinal direction. Nonapneic snorers had upper airway shapes intermediate between these two groups. Using CT scanning, Schwab et al.[28] published similar findings. These results are consistent with reports that the upper airway collapses laterally during sleep, when viewed endoscopically or by fast CT.[46] Whether the longitudinal orientation of the pharynx in patients with OSA is secondary to lateral encroachment by fat, that is, an increase in Ptis, to pharyngeal dilator muscles pulling the airway anteriorly, or both is unknown. However as mentioned above, this anteroposterior orientation could diminish the ability of pharyngeal muscles to dilate the upper airway (i.e., decreased Pmusc). [29]

Several measures have been used to evaluate the compliance or collapsibility of the human upper airway, including acoustic reflection techniques that measure the lung volume-related change in pharyngeal area, nasopharyngeal resistance, and the critical closing pressure of the airway (Pcrit). Pcrit is the PL at which the cross-sectional area of the upper airway becomes zero. Regardless of the technique used, numerous studies have suggested that fat surrounding the human upper airway increases the compliance of the pharynx.[13,32–34,51,52] This increased compliance or collapsibility could result from a direct effect on the airway itself or an indirect effect on the function of the upper airway dilator muscles (i.e., decreased Pmusc).

Obesity can also result in decreased lung volume, secondary to a decreased tendency of the chest wall to spring out, which is due to accumulation of adipose tissue in and around the ribs, abdomen and diaphragm.[53] Because the pharyngeal area is directly proportional to lung volume, and resistance and compliance inversely proportional to lung volume, obesity can decrease the baseline area and increase the resistance and compliance of the upper airway simply by its effect on lung volume.[31–34]

Obesity can also impact the degree of oxyhemoglobin desaturation and hypercapnia associated with a given abnormal respiratory event by several mechanisms: 1) increased baseline oxygen and consumption and carbon dioxide production; 2) decreased lung volume, which increases mismatch of ventilation and perfusion from airway closure and collapse (atelectasis); the result is decreased oxygen stores in the lung, decreased mixed venous oxygen saturation, and a lower baseline oxyhemoglobin saturation.[54–56] Thus, for a given abnormal respiratory event, an obese individual is more likely than his nonobese counterpart to have oxyhemoglobin desaturation and hypercapnia.

Neck circumference is a simple clinical measurement that reflects obesity in the region of the upper airway. Studies have indicated that patients with OSA have larger necks than nonapneic snorers as well as weight-matched controls.[57, 58] This parameter is related to obesity, apnea severity, tongue and soft palate size, as well as maxillary, mandibular and hyoid bone position, all thought to be important in the pathogenesis of OSA.[43,59–64] In addition, of all the anthropomorphic measurements, including BMI, the neck circumference, particularly if adjusted for height, was the strongest predictor of sleep-disordered breathing.[57,65] Waist-to-hip ratio, another measure of central obesity, also exhibits a better correlation with OSA severity than BMI.[66] These findings suggest that it is the distribution of fat, in particular upper body obesity, rather than total body fat, that is important to the development of OSA. In one study, only neck circumference and retroglossal space were independent correlates of apnea severity.[67] Nonetheless, although a more useful predictor of OSA than BMI and other signs and symptoms, neck circumference alone, even if corrected for height, is neither sufficiently sensitive nor specific to avoid the need for further diagnostic testing to establish the diagnosis (r^2 = 0.38; sensitivity = 87%; specificity = 79%; positive predictive value = 66%).[65]

Obesity Hypoventilation Syndrome

The precise underlying pathophysiology of OHS is unclear and likely multifactorial in nature, with evidence to support: (1) an impaired central drive to breath; (2) respiratory muscle fatigue, due to ventilatory muscle dysfunction and/or increased work of breathing; (3) abnormal respiratory load compensation; and (4) coexistent obstructive lung disease as possible contributors. Although the majority of individuals with OHS have OSA, the exact contribution of obstructive sleep-disordered breathing is unclear (Table 2).

Data supporting the role of abnormal ventilatory drive in OHS is mixed. Numerous studies have demonstrated reduced hypercapnic ventilatory responsiveness in OHS patients.[18,68–70] Coexistent OSA may play a role in this impaired ventilatory drive, since it is decreased in obese OSA patients compared with obese patients without OSA.[69] In addition, some patients with OHS are able to voluntarily hyperventilate to a normal arterial $PaCO_2$. This finding implies an abnormal ventilatory drive, since chest wall and lung mechanics alone can not ex-

---

Table 2
Potential Pathophysiologic Factors
in Obesity Hypoventilation Syndrome

Impaired central drive to breath
Respiratory muscle fatigue
● Increased work of breathing
    ● Decreased chest wall and lung compliance
    ● Increased chest wall, upper airway, and total system resistance
    ● Increased inspiratory threshold load
    ● Coexistent OSA or UARS
● Decreased ventilatory muscle strength and efficiency
Abnormal ventilatory load compensation
Coexistent chronic obstructive pulmonary disease

---

plain the chronic hypercapnia.[71] In contrast, Lopata et al. demonstrated that eucapnic patients with OSA and patients with OHS had similar central nervous system (CNS) drives (P.1) and diaphragmatic electromyogram (EMG) responses to progressive hypercapnia.[72] Moreover, the blunted hypercapnic response found in patients with OHS could be secondary to the compensatory elevation of serum bicarbonate (HCO_3), which confounds interpretation of these data.[73] Finally, that some OHS patients return to eucapnia after treatment with either nasal continuous positive airway pressure (CPAP) or tracheostomy, without a change in hypercapnic responsiveness, suggests that some abnormality other than or in addition to diminished ventilatory drive is playing a role.[18]

Clearly, patients with OHS are at risk for respiratory muscle fatigue, which also can result in hypercapnia. Respiratory muscle fatigue will occur if work of breathing is excessive and/or respiratory muscles operate inefficiently. Those factors that have been shown to increase work and energy cost of breathing in patients with OHS include decreased chest wall and lung compliance, the latter due in part to increased pulmonary blood volume and increased closure of dependent airways; increased chest wall, upper airway and total respiratory system resistance; increased respiratory effort against on occluded upper airway, if OSA or UARS coexists; and increased inspiratory threshold load, due to increased weight pressing on the thorax and abdomen.[74–77] Inspiratory threshold load is the load that the respiratory muscles must overcome before inspiratory flow can begin. Ventilatory muscle strength and efficiency are impaired in severe obesity, an overstretched diaphragm contributing to this diminished capacity.[79,80] Evidence to support the role of ventilatory muscle fatigue in the pathogenesis of OHS was provided by Rochester and Enson,[76] who observed that weight loss increased maximum voluntary ventilation (MVV), forced vital capacity (FVC) and reduced $PaCO_2$, despite little change in compliance of the chest wall and lungs. In addition, significant improvement in hypercapnic ventilatory responsiveness may occur within 24 hours of initiating positive pressure ventilation (PPV), the rapidity of response most consistent with relief of respiratory muscle fatigue.[81]

Ventilatory load compensation, which is the normal response taken to defend alveolar ventilation when mechanical impediments are placed on the respiratory system, is impaired in OSA, compared with weight-matched controls.[82,83] This abnormal response to elastic and resistive loads may play a role in the development of hypercapnia in patients with OSA and OHS as well.

Finally, like patients with OHS, patients with chronic obstructive pulmonary disease (COPD) have an increased energy cost and work of breathing, due to airflow obstruction and increased dead space to tidal volume ratio (Vd/Vt).[84–88] This increased Vd/Vt is secondary to parenchymal lung disease as well as the rapid shallow breathing pattern adopted by patients with COPD. In addition, patient's with COPD also have decreased respiratory muscle efficiency due to decreased blood supply to the respiratory muscles and to dynamic hyperinflation flattening the diaphragm's normal dome-shaped configuration.[88–91] As mentioned above, this combination of excessive work of breathing and inefficient ventilatory muscles increases the likelihood of respiratory muscle fatigue. Also, there is some evidence for decreased carbon dioxide (CO_2) responsiveness in patients with COPD.[92,93] Consequently, coexistent COPD would be expected to contribute to hypercapnia in obese individuals by any of the above mechanisms.

Regarding the role of OSA in the pathogenesis of OHS, Sullivan and colleagues[94] have suggested an explanation for the link between these two disorders. These investigators hypothesize that depressed chemoresponsiveness and ventilatory responses to resistive loads, and increased arousal thresholds initially serve as a protective adaptation to chronic hypoxia, hypercapnia, and sleep fragmentation. The consequence of this reduced responsiveness is less respiratory effort during inspiration. Studies have demonstrated that the arousal from sleep that opens the upper airway and terminates an apnea or hypopnea is much more tightly linked to the tension generated by the diaphragm and the time this tension is generated (tension time index) than oxyhemoglobin desaturation.[95,96] Because the tension-time index of the diaphragm is an indicator of ventilatory effort, the consequence of diminished inspiratory effort during sleep is fewer arousals from sleep. The result is reduced ventilation, also called hypoventilation, rather than no ventilation, i.e., apnea. And episodic hypopneas, apneas and arousals from sleep are replaced by hypoventilation, with its relatively unwavering hypoxemia and hypercapnia. In addition, this decreased responsiveness, combined with the increased energy expenditure of breathing, and the inefficient, sometimes fatigued muscles of massively obese individuals, results in an inability to recover between apneic periods with the normal compensatory hyperventilation response.[68] This worsens the blood gas abnormalities even further, and a vicious cycle, whereby chronic hypoxemia and hypercarbia further impair chemoresponsiveness, load compensation and arousal thresholds ensues.

Interestingly, a common feature of those patients with daytime hypercapnia and OSA is a greater degree of oxyhemoglobin desaturation during sleep, compared with eucapnic OSA patients.[97,98] This finding, as well as the improvement in ventilatory responses to both resistive loads and hypercapnia that occurs after treatment of OSA with nasal CPAP, provide supportive evidence for this theory.[81,83]

Physiological Consequences

Sleep-disordered breathing leads to arousal from sleep, oxyhemoglobin desaturation, and hypercapnia. The consequences of these abnormalities are listed in Tables 3 and 4. Although daytime sleepiness, fatigue, irritability, and personality change have been attributed to both nocturnal oxyhemoglobin desaturation and to the chronic sleep deprivation caused by sleep fragmentation, arousal from sleep is con-

Table 3
Consequences of Arousal from Sleep

- Sleep fragmentation
  - Excessive daytime sleepiness
  - Personality changes
  - Intellectual deterioration
  - Visual motor incoordination
  - Impotence
- Insomnia
- Restlessness
- Choking, gagging, gasping, resuscitative snorting

Table 4
Consequences of Nocturnal Hypoxia/hypercapnia

- Polycythemia
- Pulmonary hypertension
- Cor Pulmonale
- Chronic hypercapnia
- Morning and nocturnal headache
- Left-sided congestive heart failure
- Cardiac dysrhythmias
- Nocturnal angina
- Diurnal systemic hypertension

sidered the more important of the two factors.[99] Daytime sleepiness and visual motor incoordination are the presumed cause of the increased rate of automobile (sevenfold) and work-related accidents in patients with OSA compared with the general population.[100] The most common cardiac dysrhythmia observed in patients with OSA is a cyclic decrease and then increase in heart rate (sinus bradytachydysrhythmia).[101,102] Other associated bradydysrhythmias include marked sinus bradycardia (<30 beats per minute), sinus arrest (> 2.5 seconds) and second degree atrioventricular block. Supraventricular paroxysmal depolarizations (SVPDs), ventricular paroxysmal depolarizations (VPDs), atrial fibrillation, atrial flutter, and ventricular tachycardia are also reported. Unless there is coexistent coronary artery disease (CAD), increased VPDs and ventricular tachycardia do not typically occur until oxyhemoglobin saturation drops to less than 60% to 65%.[103,104]

Patients with sleep-disordered breathing may present with all, or only a few of the symptoms and signs listed in Tables 3 and 4. Whether an individual presents with snoring, symptoms of sleep fragmentation, signs of hypoxemia/hypercarbia or a combination, depends on several factors (Figure 8). As has already been mentioned, everything begins with some predisposing abnormality or abnormalities of the upper airway. When this predisposing factor(s) is combined with the decreased pharyngeal dilator muscle activity and lung volume that accompanies sleep onset, some degree of upper airway narrowing occurs. If the soft portions of the oro and nasopharynx vibrate, snoring will also result. Depending on the degree of narrowing and resultant increase in upper airway resistance, ventilatory effort may increase to maintain the required ventilation. Because increased ventilatory effort is transmitted to the upper airway in the form of a greater negative intra-PL, the pharynx will become narrower, further increasing upper airway resistance, and a viscous cycle may ensue.

As mentioned above, the arousal from sleep that terminates an apnea or hypopnea is much more tightly linked to increasing ventilatory effort, than oxyhemoglobin desaturation. If this "ventilatory effort arousal threshold" is exceeded while the respiratory muscles are still able to compensate for the increased upper airway resistance or load and maintain normal airflow, an arousal from sleep alone will occur. And without diminished airflow, no oxyhemoglobin desaturation or hypercapnia will result. This condition, which is associated with daytime fatigue, tiredness, and sleepiness due to the sleep fragmentation induced by the arousals, has been termed the UARS (see Definitions above).[23] Treatment with sufficient nasal CPAP pressure to eliminate the progressively increasing negative swings in intrapleural pressure

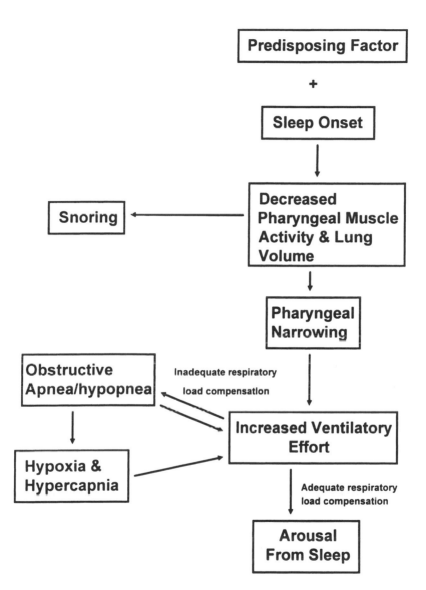

Figure 8. Pathophysiology of obstructive sleep apnea.

and the associated arousals, eliminates the daytime symptoms. Interestingly, several patients with UARS, all women, did not even snore.

If ventilatory effort does not exceed its "arousal threshold" prior to the respiratory muscles becoming unable to compensate for the increased upper airway resistance or load, a decrease in airflow and tidal volume, that is, a hypopnea results. If airflow ceases completely prior to arousal from sleep, an apnea occurs.

There are two possible outcomes of a hypopnea and apnea: a further increase in ventilatory effort followed by an arousal alone, or hypoxia and hypercapnia, which independently, as well as by further increasing ventilatory effort, usually result in an arousal from sleep. The determinants of whether an apnea or hypopnea result in oxyhemoglobin desaturation and hypercapnia, as well as the severity of these abnormalities if they do occur, is discussed above.

Finally, if the both the "ventilatory effort arousal threshold" and an individual's ability to compensate for hypoxia, hypercapnia and respiratory loads are sufficiently blunted, hypoventilation alone, without the periodic arousals that terminate hypopneas, apneas or increased upper airway resistance results.

Thus, the term OSA is not, strictly speaking, applicable to the entire spectrum of sleep-disordered breathing, but is best reserved for those individuals with the most severe form of the disease. The term obstructive sleep-disordered breathing syndrome (OSDB) better describes the entire spectrum of obstructive breathing abnormalities during sleep (Figure 9). On one end of the continuum of increased upper airway resistance is primary, asymptomatic snoring. This is followed by the UARS, then by the sleep hypopnea syndrome and finally by the sleep apnea syndrome. The OHS is used to describe individuals with OSDB who also have daytime hypoventilation and who are typically morbidly obese. The major factors that determine where along the spectrum of OSDB a patient lies are the degree of pharyngeal narrowing or upper airway resistance, the "ventilatory effort arousal threshold" and the resistive load compensation. Whether hypoventilation, a hypopnea or an apnea eventuates in hypoxia and hypercapnia depends on the duration of the abnormal respiratory event, whether the event is obstructive or central, as well as the individual's lung volume, mixed venous oxygen saturation, and baseline arterial oxygen saturation. The length of the abnormal breathing event is determined primarily by the ventilatory effort arousal threshold.

Regarding some of the other long-term consequences of OSDB, in several retrospective studies, where adjustments were made for other risk factors such as weight, age, smoking and sex, both OSA syndrome

Upper Airway Resistance

	Snoring	Arousal	Hypopnea	Apnea
UA Vibration	Yes	Yes/No	Yes/No	Yes/No
Ventilatory Effort Arousal Threshold Exceeded	No	Yes	No	No
Adequate Respiratory Load Compensation	Yes	Yes	No	No
Clinical Syndrome	Primary Snoring	UARS	Sleep Hypopnea Syndrome	Sleep Apnea Syndrome

Figure 9. Spectrum of obstructive sleep-disordered breathing syndrome. UA = upper airway; UARS = upper airway resistance syndrome. The degree of resultant hypoxemia and hypercapnia depends on the patient's underlying cardiopulmonary function (I.e. arterial and mixed venous oxyhemoglobin saturation, lung volumes) and the duration of the abnormal respiratory event. If daytime hypercapnia is present and the patient morbidly obese, the term OHS is used.

and snoring were associated with increased prevalence of hypertension, CAD and cerebral vascular accidents.[2,105] In fact, unrecognized sleep apnea occurs in approximately 20% to 30% of hypertensive patients in the United States.[106] That snoring alone is associated with increased cardiovascular morbidity suggests that even mild degrees of sleep-disordered breathing may have adverse health effects. Finally, in yet another retrospective study, He et al.[5], demonstrated that untreated significant OSA, defined as an AI greater than 20, was associated with excess mortality. Because current morbidity and mortality data is based on retrospective studies, the true impact of sleep-disordered breathing on society remains unknown. A randomized trial is clearly required, and in fact, is presently ongoing.

The mechanism whereby sleep-disordered breathing increases the risk of cardiovascular disease and consequences is unclear. It appears to be mediated by a complex interaction between the mechanical effects of repetitive increased upper airway resistance, the often associated hypoxia and hypercapnia, and their effect on the autonomic nervous system.[106]

Diagnosis

The possibility of sleep-disordered breathing should be considered in any patient with any of the predisposing factors, signs, or symptoms mentioned above (Tables 1, 3, and 4). Those symptoms and signs that have been shown to be most useful in determining the need for further diagnostic evaluation are listed in Table 5. Talking with the bed partner, family members, friends or fellow employees can be very helpful, as they will often notice signs such as apneas or falling asleep unintentionally, that the patient may be unaware of or deny. The next step is to estimate a clinical likelihood or pretest probability of sleep-disordered breathing based on a focused history and physical examination. This evaluation should include searching for alternative explanations for symptoms such as insufficient sleep or shift work causing excessive daytime sleepiness. Symptoms of excessive daytime sleepiness, unrefreshing or nonrestorative sleep, morning headaches, cognitive impairment, depression, nocturnal esophageal reflux (due to increases in abdominal pressure during upper airway obstruction), nocturia or enuresis (due to increased intraabdominal pressure

---

Table 5
Features Most Useful in Determining the Probability
of Obstructive Sleep Disordered Breathing

- Male sex
- Age >40
- Habitual snoring
- Nocturnal gasping, choking, or resuscitative snorting
- Witnessed apnea
- BMI >25 kg/m2, or neck circumference ≥17 inches in males, ≥16 inches in females
- Systemic hypertension

---

and/or secretion of atrial natriuretic hormone), hearing loss, automatic behavior, sleep drunkenness (disorientation, confusion upon awakening), hypnogogic hallucinations and night sweats, although commonly reported, do not distinguish sleep apnea from other non-pulmonary sleep disorders.

In any patient presenting with a complaint of excessive daytime sleepiness, the degree of sleepiness should be quantitated. The sleepier the individual, the more likely he has sleep-disordered breathing or some other significant disorder, and the more severe the condition, the latter influencing treatment (see below). A reasonable approach is to divide sleepiness into mild, moderate and severe, based on the frequency of sleep episodes, the degree of impairment of social and occupational function, and in what situations sleep episodes occur.[107] With mild sleepiness, sleep episodes are infrequent, may not occur every day, and occur at times of rest or when little attention is required, such as while watching TV, reading or traveling as a passenger. Sleepiness is considered severe when it is present daily, and when sleep episodes occur even during activities requiring sustained attention such as eating, conversation, walking and driving. Moderate sleepiness lies somewhere in between these extremes. Table 6 presents those sleep-inducing situations most commonly reported by patients with OSA syndrome.

It is important to remember that although the majority of patients with sleep disordered breathing are sleepy, when objectively measured by the MSLT(see Definitions above), daytime sleepiness is under reported.[108, 109] Fatigue may be the only symptom mentioned. This situation likely results because sleep-disordered breathing develops over a

---

Table 6
Sleep-inducing Situations in Apnea Patients[181]*

Situation	Percentage of Patients
Watching television	91
Reading	85
Riding in a car	71
Church	57
Visiting friends and relatives	54
Driving	50
Working	43
Waiting at a red light	32

*n = 385 patients.

long period, and patients adapt their lifestyles to compensate for it. In addition, sleepiness may be denied because of lack of awareness of risk, embarrassment, or concern regarding punitive actions such as loss of occupation.[110] Thus, the absence of sleepiness can not be used to reliably exclude OSA. In addition, sleep-disordered breathing is not the only cause of excessive daytime sleepiness (EDS), the differential diagnosis of which is depicted on Table 7. That is, EDS is not specific for sleep-disordered breathing either.

Those physical examination findings that significantly increase the likelihood of sleep-disordered breathing are listed in Table 5. Other features that should be searched for include craniofacial and upper airway abnormalities such as retrognathia; tonsillar hypertrophy, especially in children; and an enlarged soft palate. The size and consistency of the tongue; presence of pharyngeal edema or abnormal reddish coloring of the pharynx; appearance of the soft palate; size, length, and position of the uvula; evidence of trauma; nares, including whether they collapse with inspiration, particularly while the patient is supine, should also be noted (Figure 4).

Unfortunately, subjective impression alone, based on history and physical examination lacks both sensitivity (52% to 78%) as well as specificity (50% to 79%).[111–114] Although plugging clinical variables into regression formulas improves these operating characteristics somewhat, (sensitivity [79% to 92%], specificity [50% to 51%]), many involve complicated mathematical formulas, which limits their usefulness.[112,114,115] Moreover even if the clinical likelihood is low, the post-test probability

---

Table 7
Differential Diagnosis of Excessive Daytime Sleepiness

- Insufficient sleep
- Central nervous system abnormality
  - Narcolepsy
  - Post-traumatic hypersomnia
  - Recurrent hypersomnia
  - Drugs
  - Depression
  - Idiopathic hypersomnia
- Circadian rhythm disorder
- Sleep fragmentation
  - Periodic limb movement disorder
  - Sleep disordered breathing
  - Medical disorders (i.e., arthritis)
  - Neurological disorders (i.e., Parkinson's disease)

---

for OSA, defined as an RDI greater than 10, still varies between 16% and 21%.[112, 115, 116] Moreover, since the criteria for the diagnosis of OSA in these studies was an RDI greater than 10 to 15, patients with symptoms secondary to UARS would have been missed, decreasing the sensitivity of clinical assessment even further. Whether a post-test probability for OSA of 16% to 21% is low enough, will depend on the threshold at which a physician is willing to accept diagnostic uncertainty. The threshold for pursuing further diagnostic testing will likely be lower in patients with severe daytime sleepiness, comorbid illnesses such as CAD, a driving accident record and certain occupations, i.e., school bus driver.

If further diagnostic testing is deemed necessary, options include a formal sleep study or polysomnogram (PSG), and a variety of portable monitoring systems. The gold standard for diagnosing sleep-disordered breathing is a PSG. Variables typically recorded include electroencephalogram (EEG), electro-oculogram (EOG) and submental EMG to stage sleep; airflow and respiratory effort to detect and diagnose hypoventilation or the type of apnea, or hypopnea; oxygen saturation; electrocardiogram (ECG); and tibialis anterior EMG, to detect periodic leg movements. To decrease the cost of PSG and facilitate treatment, a split night study can be performed. With a split night study, the initial portion of the evening is spent determining whether sleep-disordered breathing is present. If sleep-disordered breathing is documented, the remainder of the night is spent finding and titrating the most effective treatment, which is usually nasal CPAP (see below) Using this approach, one night is required for both diagnosis and treatment, the latter adequate 60% of the time, and accepted by the patient 62% to 75% of the time.[117–119] This acceptance rate is somewhat lower than that seen with full night nasal CPAP titrations (71% to 92%).[120,121]

Because of the cost and frequent unavailability of PSG, investigators have sought less expensive alternatives to formal sleep studies performed in sleep laboratories. These portable recording devices differ in the number and types of parameters measured, varying from pulse oximetry alone, to all those variables measured in the sleep laboratory. Each is associated with its own advantages as well as disadvantages. Advantages of these portable systems include lower cost, greater availability, and they can be performed in the patient's home. Of those devices that have been studied and the results published in peer reviewed journals, their sensitivities vary from 78% to 100%, and specificity 67% to 100%, depending on the particular system, the number of variables monitored and the definition of sleep apnea.[122]

The major disadvantage of portable systems and pulse oximetry is the possibility of false-negative results. The likelihood of a false-negative study depends on the number of variables monitored, and is due to not staging sleep, observing body position, or detecting UARS. Consequently, a negative result may be a true-negative, or a false-negative secondary to the patient not falling asleep or sleeping much; not entering REM-sleep, the stage of sleep during which sleep-disordered breathing is most likely to occur; not sleeping in the supine position, the position in which sleep-disordered breathing is most likely to occur; or missing UARS. In addition, these systems can not diagnose other etiologies of excessive sleepiness such as periodic leg movements and narcolepsy. Finally, even if these portable systems were 100% specific, a formal PSG is still required if significant sleep-disordered breathing is documented. The optimum nasal CPAP pressure must be determined, and at least at the present time, this is only done in a sleep laboratory. However with the advent of Auto-CPAP devices, some of which have the capability of diagnosing sleep-disordered breathing as well as initiating treatment, this situation may soon change.

Thus, at the present time, based on the literature to date, in particular, the studies by Crocker et al. and Series et al., the following is a reasonable approach to the diagnosis of obstructive sleep-disordered breathing (Figure 10): (1) Consider the diagnosis of sleep-disordered breathing in anyone with any predisposing factor sign or symptom consistent with the diagnosis; (2) Estimate a clinical likelihood or pre-test probability based on the number and predictive value of the patient's signs and symptoms and predisposing factors, as well as the presence of alternative explanations, i.e., insufficient sleep or shift work as the cause of their daytime sleepiness; (3) Take into account the potential consequences of missing the diagnosis. That is, have a lower threshold for pursuing the diagnosis in a school bus driver, someone who has already had an auto accident, or someone with underlying CAD.[115,123]

All individuals who complain of excessive daytime sleepiness without another obvious explanation such as insufficient sleep, should undergo a split night PSG. If the overnight PSG shows no obvious etiology such as OSA or periodic limb movement disorder, a MSLT (see Definitions above) should be performed.

If the patient is not hypertensive, has a BMI less than 25 kg/m^2, and there are no witnessed apneas, the likelihood of having OSA is very low, and if excessive daytime sleepiness is not present, no screening or PSG studies are required.[115]

If the patient is not hypertensive, has no witnessed apneas, but BMI is greater than 25 kg/m^2, the probability of significant OSA is low, and nocturnal pulse oximetry should be performed. As per Series' study,

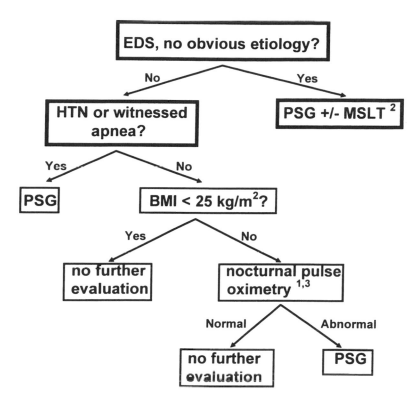

Figure 10. Diagnostic algorithm for obstructive sleep-disordered breathing syndrome. EDS = excessive daytime sleepiness; HTN = hypertension; PSG = polysomnogram; MSLT = multiple sleep latency test; BMI = body mass index. [1] Also consider diagnosis of sleep-disordered breathing and nocturnal pulse oximetry for unexplained hypercapnia, polycythemia, pulmonary hypertension and cor pulmonale. [2] Perform MSLT if no obvious etiology of EDS on PSG (i.e. significant sleep-disordered breathing, periodic limb movements). [3] See text for details of normality and abnormality.

a positive oximetry study is defined as one with a pattern of repetitive, short duration oxyhemoglobin desaturation.[123] No absolute (i.e. ≤90%) or relative (i.e., ≥ 3% to 4%) decrease in oxyhemoglobin saturation is used. With this criteria, the negative predictive value of nocturnal pulse oximetry is quite good (96.9%), but the positive predictive value is not (61.4%). Consequently, every abnormal oximetry requires follow-up. Finally, for any other constellation of signs or symptoms, perform a split night PSG.

The diagnosis of sleep-disordered breathing, which includes both

OHS and OSDB, should also be considered in any individual with unexplained daytime hypercapnia, polycythemia, pulmonary hypertension or cor-pulmonale. Patients with hypercapnia and pulmonary hypertension secondary to COPD typically have a forced expiratory volume in 1 second (FEV1) less than 1 to 1.3 L/min (30% of predicted).[124] Pulmonary hypertension predictably occurs in COPD when arterial oxygen tension PaO_2 is less than 50 mm Hg and $PaCO_2$ greater than 45 mm Hg.[125, 126] Those with pulmonary hypertension due to restrictive lung disease usually have an FVC less than 50% of predicted.[127] With systemic sclerosis, a diffusing capacity (DLCO) less than 43% was a better predictor of pulmonary hypertension than FVC less than 50%, having a sensitivity of 67%.[128]

Treatment

The optimum therapy for sleep-disordered breathing depends on the severity of disease. Consequently, the first task is to estimate this severity. Presently, the upper limit of normality for the number of sleep-disordered breathing events is an AI of 5.[129] However, such a measure does not take into account hypopneas or EEG arousals from sleep due to increased upper airway resistance alone. Furthermore, recent evidence suggests that present definitions of arousal from sleep, which are based on changes in EEG frequency and have a 3-second duration requirement, miss many arousals, which can be detected by other means such as monitoring blood pressure changes.[130] Finally, because there are no prospective studies, the clinical importance of an AI greater than 5, or any particular cutoff for normality is unclear, particularly in the elderly.[131]

Although the smallest number of arousals from sleep needed to induce a complaint is unknown, a reasonable cutoff point, based on the existing sleep fragmentation literature, is 10 per hour.[23,132,133] Thus, at the present time, it is reasonable to define OSDB as an AI greater than 5, RDI greater than 10, or greater than 10 arousals per hour of sleep due to UARS plus some physiological consequence such as excessive daytime sleepiness. Since patients with OHS may not have discrete hypopneas or apneas, such measures would not be useful in this situation. Consequently, it is important to also monitor the following parameters to help diagnose as well as determine the clinical significance and severity of sleep-disordered breathing: maximum oxyhemoglobin desaturation, presence of cardiac dysrhythmias, and daytime sleepiness,

Table 8
Severity Scale for Sleep Disordered Breathing

Severity	Respiratory Disturbance Index (RDI)	Minimum Oxygen Saturation	Cardiac Dysrhythmia	Excessive Daytime Sleepiness (EDS) MSLT (min)	ESS
Mild	> 5–15	≥ 85%	tachy-bradycardia	8–10	> 10–12
Moderate	16–30	65–84%	severe tachy-bradycardia	5–8	12–16
Severe	31–50	< 65%	ventricular tachycardia; sinus arrest or pause > 3 seconds	< 5	> 16

Table 9
Treatment of Obstructive Sleep Disordered Breathing

CONSERVATIVE	MEDICAL	SURGICAL
Weight loss	First-line	Nasal surgery
Avoid sleep deprivation	Nasal positive airway	Upper airway reconstruction
Avoid alcohol	pressure	Adenotonsillectomy
Avoid sedative-hypnotics	CPAP	Uvulopalatopharyngoplasty
Positional therapy	Bilevel	Laser-assisted
Treat nasal congestion	Nasal volume ventilation	uvulopalatoplasty
Treat hypothyroidism	Second-line	Maxillofacial surgery
Treat acromegaly	Oral appliance	Inferior sagital mandibular
	Other	osteotomy +
	Medications	genioglossal
	Fluoxetine, protryptyline,	advancement +/− hyoid
	medroxyprogesterone,	myotomy and suspension
	acetazolamide	Maxillomandibular
	Nocturnal oxygen	osteotomy and
	Mask or nasal cannula	advancement
	Transtracheal	Tongue reduction surgery
		Laser midline glossectomy
		Upper airway bypass
		Tracheostomy
		Bariatric surgery
		Gastric bypass
		Jejeuno-ileal bypass
		Gastroplasty

defined either objectively by MSLT or subjectively by a measure such as the Epworth sleepiness scale.[134] The severity scale I typically use is depicted on Table 8.

The goals of treatment are the elimination of all evidence of increased upper airway resistance, which includes apneas, hypopneas, and UARS; an oxyhemoglobin saturation 88% to 90% or less; elimination of sleep disruption due to UARS, hypopneas or apneas; and the elimination of snoring.

Therapeutic options for sleep-disordered breathing can be divided into conservative, medical and surgical (Table 9).

Conservative Treatment

Although the importance of avoiding factors that can increase the severity of sleep-disordered breathing should be discussed with all patients, if the patient has mild disease and a clear predisposing factor conservative therapy may be all that is required. Patients should avoid factors that can increase the severity of upper airway resistance such as sleep deprivation, alcohol and sedative-hypnotic agents.[135–138] Sleep deprivation increases upper airway hypotonia and delays contraction of pharyngeal dilator muscles.[139] Both alcohol and sedative-hypnotic agents increase the frequency of abnormal breathing events during sleep by reducing upper airway muscle tone and prolonging abnormal respiratory events by increasing the arousal threshold.[136–138] In some individuals, sleep-disordered breathing occurs only in the supine position. Training individuals to sleep primarily in the supine position, i.e., with a tennis ball attached to the nightshirt, may completely alleviate their sleep-disordered breathing , though the long-term effectiveness of this intervention is unclear.[140] If present, treatment of increased nasal resistance with a combination of nasal steroids, decongestants and/or antihistamines should be undertaken. Likewise, hypothyroidism and acromegaly should be treated appropriately. Because treatment of hypothyroidism without concomitant treatment of OSA may result in more severe oxyhemoglobin desaturation due to increased oxygen consumption, both should be treated concurrently (ie, with nasal CPAP). Nasal CPAP treatment may be discontinued after treatment of the endocrine abnormality, if a follow-up PSG no longer demonstrates significant sleep-disordered breathing.

In obese individuals with OSA, dietary weight loss can significantly decrease the number of abnormal respiratory events, oxyhemoglobin desaturation, sleep fragmentation, daytime performance, and cardiovascular and pulmonary function.[141–143] Unfortunately, there is no information on the amount of weight loss needed to achieve improvement.

That is, it is not known if a critical threshold of weight loss exists. There is also no long-term follow-up on the maintenance of the weight loss and improvement in sleep-disordered breathing, although other sources suggest that a high degree of relapse is to be expected.[144,145]

Medical Treatment

Nasal Continuous Positive Airway Pressure

For patients with moderate to severe disease, conservative treatment alone is rarely adequate, and treatment with nasal CPAP becomes the next therapeutic option. With this device, CPAP is applied to the upper airway with a nasal mask, nasal prongs, or an oronasal mask.[146-2D148] Although there are numerous proposed mechanisms, CPAP acts predominantly by providing a "positive pressure or pneumatic splint" to the upper airway, preventing the airway narrowing that occurs when dilator muscle activity decreases at sleep onset (Figure 11). CPAP has been shown to completely reverse or at least significantly improve all of the symptoms due to sleep fragmentation and oxyhemoglobin desaturation and hypercapnia mentioned above, including diurnal hypertension, daytime hypercapnia, pulmonary hypertension and cor pulmonale.[146, 149]

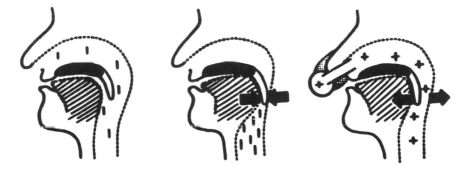

Figure 11. Schematic representation of the effect of CPAP on the upper airway in obstructive sleep apnea. The **top panel** demonstrates that negative airway pressure is generated during inspiration and that muscle tone is needed to prevent airway collapse. The **middle panel** represents airway occlusion resulting form negative intra-airway pressure exceeding muscle forces tending to maintain airway patency. The **lower panel** shows the theoretical effect of reversing the negative airway pressure with continuous positive pressure. (From Martin RJ: Medical treatment for the sleep apnea syndrome. In Fletcher EC (ed): *Abnormalities of Respiration During Sleep.* Orlando, Fl, Grune & Stratton, Inc, 1986, p. 105, with permission.)

In patients with OHS, including those associated with OSDB, therapy with nasal CPAP may be ineffective or only partially effective. In such individuals, significant oxyhemoglobin desaturation and hypercapnia persist, particularly during REM-sleep, despite the absence or elimination of upper airway obstruction and the addition of supplemental oxygen. In such situations, the patient requires either supplemental oxygen, or ventilation with a nasal bilevel system or a nasal volume ventilator with or without supplemental oxygen (see below).

If tolerated, nasal CPAP is effective in the majority of cases of obstructive sleep-disordered breathing. Thus, the major limiting factor is compliance, with subjective estimates by the patient being much higher than objective measurements. In one study, only 46% of patients complied with treatment, with compliance being defined rather loosely as wearing the CPAP machine for 4 hours or more on 70% or more of the nights.[150] Compliance appears more closely linked to the relief of daytime symptoms such as decreased alertness than to the severity of the RDI.[146]

At least part of the reason for the poor compliance is side effects, which can be divided into nasopharyngeal and pressure-related symptoms. The inconvenience of being attached to a machine is also a problem. Although the precise cause of the nasopharyngeal symptoms is unknown, they likely result from the machine's cool, dry air injuring the lining epithelium and/or stimulating nerves in the nasopharynx. Tables 10 and 11 list the potential adverse effects, as well as recommended treatment. The function of the ramp option found on most CPAP machines is to allow the CPAP pressure to gradually increase to the prescribed level over a period of 5 to 45 minutes.

Table 10
Adverse Effects of Nasal CPAP

Nasopharyngeal symptoms	Pressure related symptoms	Other
Congestion (20%)	Chest wall discomfort ($< 5\%$)	Mouth opening
Dry nose/mouth (25%)	Ear discomfort	Claustrophobia
Sinus discomfort (10%)	Difficult exhaling	Conjunctivitis
Headache	Can't fall asleep	Bridge of nose
Ear discomfort/infection	Awakens smothering	bruise/ulceration
Epistaxis	Barotrauma	Allergic reaction
	Pneumothorax	
	Pneumomediastinum	
	Pneumoencephalus	

Table 11
Treatment of Adverse Effects of Nasal CPAP

Nasopharyngeal Symptoms	Pressure Related Symptoms	Mouth Opening	Claustrophobia	Conjunctivitis	Bridge of Nose Bruise/Ulceration	Allergic Reaction
Humidification	Ramp	Chin strap	Different mask	Adjust mask fit	Reinforce area	Different mask
Nasal salt solution/spray	BiPAP	Form fitting mouth guard	Relaxation techniques	Different mask	Different mask	
Add humidifier to machine	Relaxation techniques	Oronasal mask	Desensitization			
Nasal steroids						
Other						
For nasal congestion						
Infrequent: alpha						
adrenergic spray						
Frequent: alpha						
adrenergic pill						
Intractable:						
oronasal mask						
For rhinorrhea						
Anticholinergic spray						
Nasal Nedocromil						
Nasal Cromolyn sodium						

Nasal Bilevel Positive Airway Pressure

Bilevel positive airway pressure (BiPAP, Respironics, Inc., Murrysville, PA.) systems differ from CPAP in that the former allows independent adjustment of inspiratory positive airway pressure (IPAP) and expiratory positive airway pressure (EPAP). With nasal CPAP, IPAP and EPAP pressures are the same. Depending on the particular bilevel machine, these systems also allow the operator to set a back-up respiratory rate, change the ratio of IPAP to EPAP time, and adjust the flow sensitivity. Thus, unlike nasal CPAP, bilevel systems permit ventilation of the patient. In addition, since a higher pressure is required to maintain adequate upper airway patency during inspiration than expiration, a bilevel system allows the EPAP pressure to be reduced. This lower EPAP pressure may diminish problems with exhaling or a smothering sensation, the risk of barotrauma (due to a lower mean alveolar pressure), and the risk of hypercapnia (since ventilation can be instituted). However, although patient acceptance may be better with bilevel systems, compliance is similar to that with CPAP.[151]

If hypercapnia persists on a nasal bilevel system, one possibility is that the patient is rebreathing exhaled CO_2. Replacing the standard exhalation device (a hole in the nasal mask) with a special non-rebreather valve, or increasing the EPAP pressure to 8 cm H_2O or morewill alleviate this situation.[152]

Nasal Volume Ventilation

In some patients with OHS with or without coexistent OSDB and COPD, chest wall impedence due to obesity may be so high that bilevel positive pressure systems may not be able to generate sufficiently high peak inspiratory pressures to correct the oxyhemoglobin desaturation and hypercapnia. In such situations a nasal volume ventilator, which can generate sufficiently high inspiratory pressures, may be required.[94]

In many patients with OHS secondary to OSDB, once the hypercapnia has improved, which typically takes 7 to 18 days, nasal CPAP may then be used.[94]

Oral Appliances[153–155]

Currently, dental appliances are considered useful for primary snoring, but second-line therapy for obstructive sleep-disordered breathing. These devices can be considered for patients with mild OSA who do not respond to conservative measures, or with moderate to severe disease if they are intolerant of, refuse, or are not candidates for nasal CPAP, a bilevel system, and surgery. Those devices that work, appear to do so by increasing the posterior airway space by providing a stable anterior position of the mandible, by advancing the tongue or soft palate, and possibly by changing genioglossus muscle activity. Close cooperation between physician and dentist is necessary to ensure optimal patient selection and follow-up, and to avoid potential side effects. Problems include tongue, gum or TMJ soreness and orthodontic problems. Compliance ranges from 50% to 100%, and in a recent study, was preferred over nasal CPAP. As for surgical procedures for OSA (see below), it is difficult to predict success, and treatment may improve OSA somewhat, but the patient is still left with significant residual disease. Consequently, a follow-up sleep study is required for moderate to severe disease, but not primary snoring or mild OSA.

Medications

Fluoxetine and tricyclic antidepressants such as protriptyline, which decrease the amount of REM sleep and increase the tone of upper airway muscles, may be useful for patients with mild OSDB who can't tolerate CPAP or lose weight.[138,156,157] These medications also may allow a decrease in high nasal CPAP pressures. Anticholinergic side effects with the tricyclic antidepressants are a significant problem.

Progestational agents such as medroxyprogesterone augment hypercapnic ventilatory chemosensitivity and resting ventilation.[158,159] These medications are not useful in the majority of patients with OSA.[160] They may have a role in patients with OHS, with or without coexistent OSA, but the data is too limited to make recommendations.[161,162]

There is also scant data on the use of acetazolamide for OSDB and OHS, which stimulates respiration by inducing a metabolic acidosis. Although effects are unpredictable, and usually small, this drug may have a role in normocapnic patients with primarily central apneas.[163–165] In addition, acetazolamide can actually induce obstructive apneas. Overall, the respiratory stimulants theophylline and almitrine are not useful for OSDB and OHS.[166]

Supplemental oxygen, administered via nasal cannula, may improve nocturnal oxyhemoglobin desaturation in patients with sleep apnea and hypoventilation. However, because it does not improve the associated sleep fragmentation and daytime sleepiness, oxygen alone is not an adequate treatment option for OSDB.[167,168]

Compared with no therapy and nasal cannula oxygen, transtracheal oxygen delivery resulted in a decrease in RDI, improved nocturnal oxygen saturation, no increase in mean apnea duration and diminished daytime sleepiness.[169] Although these findings suggest that transtracheal oxygen may be a safe and effective alternative treatment of OSA, data is too sparse to make strong recommendations.

The role of anorexiant drugs such as fenfluramine and phentermine in the treatment of OSA is also unclear. In one uncontrolled study with 13 patients over 6 months, fenfluramine resulted in a decreased, though still markedly abnormal RDI, and a reduction of required nasal CPAP pressures.[170] Clearly, additional trials with anorexiant drugs in the treatment of sleep-disordered breathing appears warranted. However, their association with primary pulmonary hypertension is a significant concern.

In summary, overall, medications are not very effective in the treatment of OSDB or OHS. With the exception, perhaps, of fluoxetine and tricyclic antidepressants in patients with mild OSDB, oxygen for central apnea and hypoventilation, and anorexiant drugs such as fenfluramine, medications for the treatment of OSDB and OHS should be limited to patients who refuse, cannot tolerate, or have contraindications to nasal positive airway pressure and surgery. Moreover when utilized, follow-up PSG in patients who appear to have responded to treatment is mandatory.

Surgical Treatment

The goal of surgery is to improve one of the determinants of upper airway caliber described above.

Nasal Surgery

Nasal surgery alone is rarely curative, but is often used in conjunction with other surgical procedures, i.e., as part of "Phase 1" surgery for OSA (see below).

Adenotonsillectomy

Although this procedure can be curative in children and adolescents with OSA, it is not usually helpful in adults.[171,172]

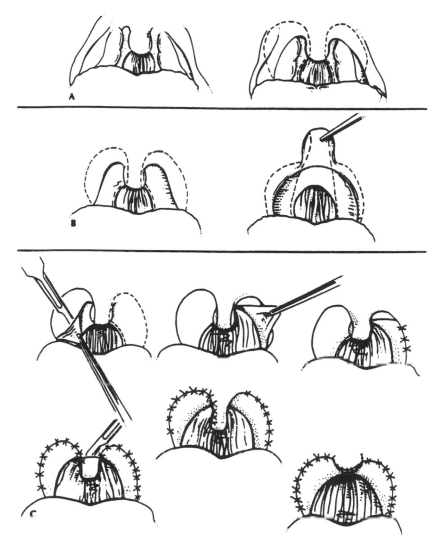

Figure 12. Uvalopalatopharyngoplasty (UPPP). Tonsillectomy is performed if it has not been done previously. If it has been done previously, the muscosa of the tonsillar fossae is excised. An incision is made in the soft palate, several millimeters lateral to the medial margin of the glossopalatal arch, extending from the inferior pole of the tonsillar fossa to the root of the uvula, then to its tip, then up the pharyngeal side of the uvula, continuing along the pharyngopalatal arch to the inferior pole of the tonsillar fossa. **A.** UPPP incisions in a patient who has not had prior tonsillectomy. **B.** UPPP incisions in a patient who has had prior tonsillectomy. **C.** Completion of UPPP in a patient who has had prior tonsillectomy. (Reproduced from Reference 172 with permission.)

Uvulopalatopharyngoplasty

The most commonly performed surgical procedure for OSDB is UPPP. The procedure involves removal of the tonsils, uvula, redundant soft palate and pharyngeal folds (Figure 12). The overall success rate is less than 50%.[173,174] Moreover, preoperative imaging studies and testing can not reliably predict surgical success.[60] This procedure is most likely to be successful if upper airway collapse is limited to the oropharynx, and the RDI less than 20 to 30, that is, with less severe disease.[177] Unfortunately, in 75% of cases, there is more than 1 site of upper airway obstruction, a fact which is the likely explanation for the poor success rate.[26] Interestingly, a recent study demonstrated that although UPPP resulted in no significant objective change in snoring or quality of sleep, subjectively, 78% of patients reported a decrease in the former, and 79% a decrease in the latter.[175] Potential complications include nasal reflux and speech problems. Postoperative pain is significant.

Laser-assisted Uvulopalatoplasty (LAUP)[176]

LAUP has recently been introduced as an outpatient treatment for snoring and potentially for obstructive sleep-disordered breathing. It involves removing part of the uvula and associated soft palate with a CO_2 laser in 1 to 7 sessions. Unlike the surgical UPPP, neither the tonsils nor the lateral pharyngeal tissues are removed or altered. Although less painful than UPPP, 60% to 75% of patients report severe postoperative pain from 1 to 8, up to 21 days. Snoring is subjectively cured or softer in 76% to 78% of cases, with best results occurring when a long uvula or a draping soft palate are present. LAUP is currently not recommended for the treatment of OSDB. However if performed for this reason, a post operative PSG is essential. One potential problem with LAUP is that the elimination of snoring removes one of the signs of OSDB, and may provide a false sense of security.

Maxillofacial Surgery[177]

Because of the poor and unpredictable results with UPPP, a variety of other procedures have been developed to further increase the size of the upper airway. Such surgeries ideally have both an otorhinolaryngologist and oral surgeon involved. Inferior sagittal mandibular osteotomy plus genioglossal advancement, with or without a hyoid myotomy and suspension enlarges the retrolingual airway (Figure 13). These proce-

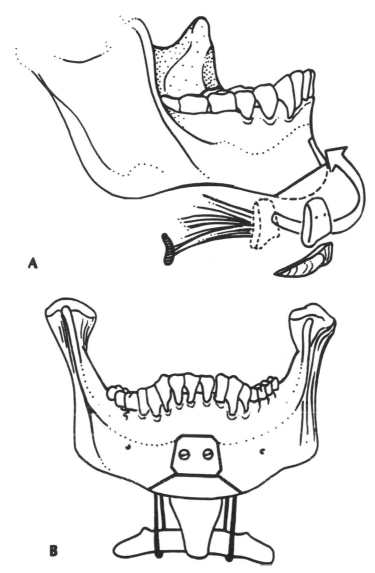

Figure 13. Genioglossal advancement with hyoid myotomy and suspension. Following a limited mandibular osteotomy, which isolates the genioid tubercle, the released segment of bone is drawn anteriorly and fixed into a position anterior to the mandible. Hyoid myotomy frees the hyoid from its inferior muscle attachments in the neck. Hyoid suspension is accomplished by passing a strip of fascia lata around the body of the hyoid and fixing it to the anterior mandible. (Note: a different technique for hyoid suspension has recently been introduced). **A.** Diagrammatic representation of the anterior movement of the freed segment of mandible with the attached genioglossus to its new position anterior to the mandible. **B.** The freed segment of mandible is fixed in position anterior to the mandible. The hyoid is freed from its inferior attachments in the neck and is suspended from the anterior mandible by strips of fascia lata. (Reproduced from Reference 172 with permission.)

dures may be performed in conjunction with a UPPP and nasal surgery. With success being defined as an RDI less than 20% and a 50% or more decrease, there is a 66% to 67% response rate to this "Phase 1" surgery.[177, 178] Complications include need for a root canal, numbness, dysesthesia of the chin for 3 to 6 months, and facial contour changes.

If the patient has significant craniofacial abnormalities and/or has not responded to "Phase 1" surgery, maxillomandibular osteotomy and advancement is an option (Figure 14). This procedure further advances the tongue and enlarges the retropalatal airway as well. In the right hands, results have been quite good, with a greater than 90% success rate being reported.[177] Average hospital stay is 2 days, the major complications being dysesthesia or paresthesia of the face that lasts 6 weeks to 6 months.

Tongue Reduction Surgery

Laser midline glossectomy is also an option for those who fail the above mentioned surgical procedures. However, this procedure is associated with a long difficult recovery, speech problems and some persistent sensory loss. The substantial associated edema requires placement of a temporary tracheostomy.

Tracheostomy

With the many surgical options, and in particular the advent of nasal CPAP and BiPAP, tracheostomy is infrequently used as treatment for OSA. This procedure should be required in less than 5% of cases. Nonetheless, there is a small subgroup of patients with severe OSDB who cannot tolerate or do not respond to other therapeutic options. In these individuals tracheostomy, which completely bypasses the upper airway obstruction, can provide dramatic improvement and be lifesaving. However, the potential for additional medical as well as psychological morbidity needs to be taken into account.[179]

Bariatric Surgery[141]

For significantly obese individuals with either OSDB or OHS, surgical weight loss procedures are another option. Weight-loss surgical procedures that have been studied include gastric bypass,

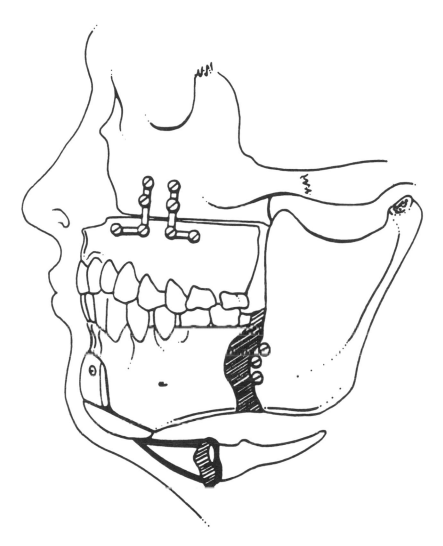

Figure 14. Maxillomandibular advancement. Mandibular and maxillary osteotomies are performed, both mandible and maxilla are advanced. Genioglossal advancement with hyoid myotomy and suspension have also been performed. (Reproduced from Reference 172 with permission.)

jejeuno-ileal bypass and gastroplasty. Results have been quite impressive and include a weight change of 31% to 72.5%, a decrease in RDI of 89% to 98%, improved nocturnal oxyhemoglobin saturation, decreased cardiac dysrhythmias, improved subjective daytime somnolence, and improved sleep continuity and architecture (increased total sleep time, % slow wave sleep, % REM sleep). Unfortunately, all studies of the effect of weight loss on sleep-disordered breathing, thus far, are poorly designed, and little more than a series of case reports. Moreover, good data on the risks and benefits of surgery, the effects of bariatric surgery on waking performance, and long-term follow-up on either the weight loss or improvements in sleep and sleep-disordered breathing are lacking. Clearly more and better controlled studies are needed.

Summary

Obesity is associated with numerous significant adverse health effects, one of which is on breathing during sleep. It is the most common predisposing factor for OSA and a requirement for OHS. Although obesity hypoventilation is an uncommon disorder, clinically significant OSA has a high prevalence, affecting 6% of the middle aged adult working population. Both disorders can present quite subtly, and are frequently overlooked. If undiagnosed, they may be associated with significant cardiovascular morbidity and even mortality. Moreover, they are readily and noninvasively diagnosed, and typically easily treated. Consequently, it would behoove all physicians to at least consider sleep-disordered breathing in any patient who has any predisposing factor, sign or symptom associated with these disease entities.

References

1. Young T, Palta M, Dempsey J, et al: The occurrence of sleep-disordered breathing among middle-aged adults. *N Engl J Med* 328:1230–1235, 1993.
2. Hung J, Whitford EG, Parsons RW, et al: Association of sleep apnea with myocardial infarction in men. *Lancet* 336:261–264, 1990.
3. Telakivi T, Partinen M, Koskenvuo M, et al: Snoring and cardiovascular disease. *Comprehens Ther* 13:53–57, 1987.
4. Partinen M, Guilleminault C: Daytime sleepiness and vascular morbidity

at seven year follow-up in obstructive sleep apnea patients. *Chest* 97:27–32, 1989.

5. He J, Kryger MH, Zorick FJ, et al: Mortality and apnea index in obstructive sleep apnea. Experience in 385 male patients. *Chest* 94:9–14, 1988.

6. Levinson PD, McGarvey ST, Carlisle CC, et al: Adiposity and cardiovascular risk factors in men with obstructive sleep apnea. *Chest* 103:1336–1342, 1993.

7. Phillips B, Cook Y, Schmitt F, et al: Sleep apnea: Prevalence of risk factors in a general population. *South Med J* 82:1090–1092, 1989.

8. Rajala R, Partinen M, Sane T, et al: Obstructive sleep apnea syndrome in morbidly obese patients. *J Intern Med* 230:125–129, 1991.

9. Dealberto MJ, Ferber C, Garma L, et al: Factors related to sleep apnea syndrome in sleep clinic patients. *Chest* 105:1753–1758, 1994.

10. Harman EM, Wynne JW, Block AJ: The effect of weight loss on sleep-disordered breathing and oxygen desaturation in morbidly obese men. *Chest* 82:291–294, 1982.

11. Smith PL, Gold AR, Meyers DA, et al: Weight loss in mildly to moderately obese patients with obstructive sleep apnea. *Ann Intern Med* 103:850–855, 1985.

12. Pasquali R, Colella P, Cirignotta F, et al: Treatment of obese patients with obstructive sleep apnea syndrome (OSAS): Effect of weight loss and interference of otorhinolaryngoiatric pathology. *Int J Obes* 14:207–217, 1990.

13. Rubinstein I, Colapinto N, Rotstein LE, et al: Improvement in upper airway function after weight loss in patients with obstructive sleep apnea. *Am Rev Respir Dis* 138:1192–1195, 1988.

14. Suratt PM, McTier RF, Findley LJ, et al: Changes in breathing and the pharynx after weight loss in obstructive sleep apnea. *Chest* 92:631–637, 1987.

15. Schwartz AR, Gold AR, Schubert N, et al: Effect of weight loss on upper airway collapsibility in obstructive sleep apnea. *Am Rev Respir Dis* 144:494–498, 1991.

16. Loube DI, Loube AA, Mitler MM: Weight loss for obstructive sleep apnea: The optimal therapy for obese patients. *J Am Diet Assoc* 94:1291–1295, 1994.

17. Martin TJ, Sanders MH: Chronic alveolar hypoventilation: A review for the clinician. *Sleep* 18:617–634, 1995.

18. Rapaport DM, Garay SM, Epstein H, et al: Hypercapnia in the obstructive sleep apnea syndrome. A reevaluation of the "Pickwickian syndrome". *Chest* 89:627–635, 1986.

19. Obstructive sleep apnea syndrome. In: *The International Classification of Sleep Disorders: Diagnostic and Coding Manual.* Rochester, American Sleep Disorders Association, 1990, pp. 52–58.

20. Gould GA, Whyte KF, Rhind GB, et al: The sleep hypopnea syndrome. *Am Rev Respir Dis* 137:895–898, 1988.

21. Moser NJ, Phillips BA, Berry DT, et al: What is hypopnea, anyway? *Chest* 105:426–428, 1994.

22. Central sleep apnea syndrome. In: *The International Classification of Sleep Disorders: Diagnostic and Coding Manual.* Rochester, American Sleep Disorders Association, 1990, pp. 58–61.

23. Guilleminault C, Stoohs R, Clerk A, et al: A cause of excessive daytime sleepiness: The upper airway resistance syndrome. *Chest* 104:781–787, 1993
24. Burwell CS, Robin ED, Whaley R, et al: Extreme obesity associated with alveolar hypoventilation. A Pickwickian syndrome. *Am J Med* 21:811, 1956.
25. Guidelines for the Multiple Sleep Latency Test (MSLT): A Standard Measure of Sleepiness. *Sleep* 9:519–524, 1986.
26. Anatomy and Physiology of upper airway obstruction. In: Kryger MH, Roth T, Dement WC (eds): *Principles and Practice of Sleep Medicine.* Philadelphia, W.B. Saunders Company, 1994, pp. 642–656.
27. Remmers JE, deGroot WJ, Sauerland EK, et al: Pathogenesis of upper airway occlusion during sleep. *J Appl Physiol* 44:931–938, 1978.
28. Schwab RJ, Gefter WB, Hoffman EA, et al: Dynamic upper airway imaging during awake respiration in normal subjects and patients with sleep disordered breathing. *Am Rev Respir Dis* 148:1385–1400, 1993.
29. Leiter JC: Upper airway shape: Is it important in the pathogenesis of obstructive sleep apnea? *Am J Respir Crit Care Med* 153:894–898, 1996.
30. Rodenstein DO, Dooms G, Thomas Y, et al: Pharyngeal shape and dimensions in healthy subjects, snorers, and patients with obstructive sleep apnea. *Thorax* 45:722–727, 1990.
31. Van de Graaff WB: Thoracic traction on the trachea: Mechanisms and magnitude. *J Appl Physiol* 70:1328–1336, 1991.
32. Brown IG, Bradley TD, Phillipson EA, et al: Pharyngeal compliance in snoring subjects with and without obstructive sleep apnea. *Am Rev Respir Dis* 132:211–215, 1985.
33. Hoffstein V, Zamel N, Phillipson EA: Lung volume dependence of pharyngeal cross-sectional area in patients with obstructive sleep apnea. *Am Rev Respir Dis* 130:175–178, 1984.
34. Brown IB, McClean PA, Boucher R, et al: Changes in pharyngeal cross-sectional area with posture and application of continuous positive airway pressure in patients with obstructive sleep apnea. *Am Rev Respir Dis* 136:628–632, 1987.
35. Shepard JWJ: Cardiorespiratory changes in obstructive sleep apnea. In: Kryger MH, Roth T, Dement WC (eds): *Principles and Practice of Sleep Medicine.* Philadelphia, W.B. Saunders Company, 1994, pp. 657–666.
36. Berger RJ: Tonus of extrinsic laryngeal muscles during sleep and dreaming. *Science* 134:840, 1961.
37. Ballard RD, Irvin CG, Martin RJ: Influence of sleep on lung volume in asthmatic patients and normal subjects. *J Appl Physiol* 68:2034–2041, 1990.
38. Wiegand DA, Latz B, Zwillich CW, et al: Geniohyoid muscle activity in normal men during wakefulness and sleep. *J Appl Physiol* 69:1262–1269, 1990.
39. Hudgel DW, Martin RJ, Johnson B, et al: Mechanics of respiratory system and breathing pattern during sleep in normal humans. *J Appl Physiol* 56:133–137, 1984.

40. Orem J: Medullary respiratory neuron activity: Relationship to tonic and phasic REM sleep. *J Appl Physiol* 48:54–65, 1980.
41. Berthon-Jones M, Sullivan CE: Ventilation and arousal responses to hypoxia in sleeping humans. *Am Rev Respir Dis* 125:632–639, 1982.
42. Douglas NJ, White DP, Weil JV, et al: Hypercapnic ventilatory response in sleeping adults. *Am Rev Respir Dis* 126:758–762, 1982.
43. Rivlin J, Hoffstein V, Kalbfleisch J, et al: Upper airway morphology in patients with idiopathic obstructive sleep apnea. *Am Rev Respir Dis* 129:355–360, 1984.
44. Horner RL, Mohiaddin RH, Lowell DG, et al: Sites and sizes of fat deposits around the pharynx in obese patients with obstructive sleep apnea and weight matched controls. *Eur Respir J* 2:613–622, 1989.
45. Shelton KE, Gay SB, Hollowell DE, et al: Mandible enclosure of upper airway and weight in obstructive sleep apnea. *Am Rev Respir Dis* 148:195–200, 1993.
46. Shelton KE, Woodson H, Gay S, et al: Pharyngeal fat in obstructive sleep apnea. *Am Rev Respir Dis* 148:462–466, 1993.
47. Stauffer JL, Buick MK, Bixler EO, et al: Morphology of the uvula in obstructive sleep apnea. *Am Rev Respir Dis* 140:724–728, 1989.
48. Schwab RJ, Gupta KB, Gefter WB, et al: Upper airway and soft tissue anatomy in normal subjects and patients with sleep-disordered breathing. Significance of the lateral pharyngeal walls. *Am Respir Crit Care Med* 152:1673–1689, 1995.
49. Listerud J, Lenkinski RE, Axel L, et al: Hydrogen ultrathin phase-encoded spectroscopy (HUPSPEC). *Magn Reson Imag* 14:507–521, 1990.
50. Schwab RJ, Prasad A, Gupta KB, et al: Fat and water measurements of the upper airway soft tissues in normal subjects and patients with sleep disordered breathing using magnetic resonance proton spectroscopy. *Am Rev Respir Dis* 145:A214, 1991.
51. Bradley TD, Brown IG, Grossman RF, et al: Pharyngeal size in snorers, nonsnorers, and patients with obstructive sleep apnea. *N Engl J Med* 315:1327–1331, 1986.
52. Rubinstein I, Hoffstein V, Bradley TD: Lung volume-related changes in the pharyngeal area of obese females with and without obstructive sleep apnea. *Eur Respir J* 2:344–351, 1989.
53. Naimark A, Cherniack RM: Compliance of the respiratory system and its components in health and obesity. *J Appl Physiol* 15:377–382, 1960.
54. Dempsey JA, Reddan W, Balke B, et al: Work capacity determinants and physiologic cost of weight-supported breathing in obesity. *J Appl Physiol* 21:1815–1820, 1966.
55. Don HG, Crain DB, Wahbo WM, et al: The measurement of gas trapped in the lungs at functional residual capacity and the effects of posture. *Anesthesiology* 35:582–590, 1971.
56. Holley HS, Milic-Emili J, Becklake MR, et al: Regional distribution of pulmonary ventilation and perfusion in obesity. *J Clin Invest* 46:475–481, 1967.
57. Katz I, Stradling J, Slutsky AS, et al: Do patients with obstructive sleep apnea have thick necks? *Am Rev Respir Dis* 141:1228–1231, 1990.
58. Hoffstein V, Mateika S: Differences in abdominal and neck circumferences

in patients with and without obstructive sleep apnea. *Eur Respir J* 5:377–381, 1992.

59. Ferguson KA, Ono T, Lowe AA, et al: The relationship between obesity and craniofacial structure in obstructive sleep apnea. *Chest* 108:375–381, 1995.

60. Shepard JWJ, Gefter WB, Guilleminault C, et al: Evaluation of the upper airway in patients with obstructive sleep apnea. *Sleep* 14:361–371, 1991.

61. deBerry-Borowiecki B, Kukwa A, Blanks RH: Cephalometric analysis for diagnosis and treatment of obstructive sleep apnea. *Laryngoscope* 98:226–234, 1988.

62. Bacon WH, Krieger J, Turlot JC, et al: Craniofacial characteristics in patients with obstructive sleep apneas syndrome. *Cleft Palate J* 25:374–378, 1988.

63. Strelzow VV, Blanks RH, Basile A, et al: Cephalometric airway analysis in obstructive sleep apnea syndrome. *Laryngoscope* 98:1149–1158, 1988.

64. Partinen M, Guilleminault C, Quera-Salva MA, et al: Obstructive sleep apnea and cephalometric roentgenograms. The role of anatomic upper airway abnormalities in the definition of abnormal breathing during sleep. *Chest* 93:1199–1205, 1988.

65. Davies RJ, Ali NJ, Stradling JR: Neck circumference and other clinical features in the diagnosis of the obstructive sleep apnea syndrome. *Thorax* 47:101–105, 1992.

66. Grunstein R, Wilcox I, Yang TS, et al: Snoring and sleep apnea in men: Association with central obesity and hypertension. *Int J Obes Relat Metab Disord* 17:533–540, 1993.

67. Davies RJ, Stradling JR: The relationship between neck circumference, radiographic pharyngeal anatomy, and the obstructive sleep apnea syndrome. *Eur Respir J* 3:509–514, 1990.

68. Garay SM, Rapoport D, Sorkin B, et al: Regulation of ventilation in the obstructive sleep apnea syndrome. *Am Rev Respir Dis* 124:451–457, 1981.

69. Gold AR, Schwartz AR, Wise RA, et al: Pulmonary function and respiratory chemosensitivity in moderately obese patients with sleep apnea. *Chest* 103:1325–1329, 1993.

70. Zwillich CW, Sutton FD, Pierson DJ, et al: Decreased hypoxic ventilatory drive in the obesity-hypoventilation syndrome. *Am J Med* 59:343–348, 1975.

71. Leech J, Onal E, Aronson R, et al: Voluntary hyperventilation in obesity hypoventilation. *Chest* 100:1334–1338, 1991.

72. Lopata M, Onal E: Mass loading, sleep apnea, and the pathogenesis of obesity hypoventilation. *Am Rev Respir Dis* 126:640–645, 1982.

73. Heinemann HO, Goldring RM: Bicarbonate and the regulation of ventilation. *Am J Med* 57:361–370, 1974.

74. Sharp JT, Henry JP, Sweany SK, et al: The total work of breathing in normal and obese men. *J Clin Invest* 43:728–739, 1964.

75. Pelosi P, Croci M, Ravagnaan I, et al: Total respiratory system, lung, and chest wall mechanics in sedated-paralyzed postoperative morbidly obese patients. *Chest* 109:144–151, 1996.

76. Rochester DF, Enson Y: Current concepts in the pathogenesis of the obesity-hypoventilation syndrome. *Am J Med* 57:402–420, 1974.

77. Suratt PM, Wilhoit S, Hsiao H, et al: Compliance of chest wall in obese subjects. *J Appl Physiol* 57:403–407, 1984.

78. Sampson MG, Grassino K: Neuromechanical properties in obese patients during carbon dioxide rebreathing. *Am J Med* 75:81–90, 1983.
79. Ray CS, Sue DY, Bray G, et al: Effects of obesity on respiratory function. *Am Rev Respir Dis* 128:501–506, 1983.
80. Berthon-Jones M, Sullivan CE: Time course of change in ventilatory response to CO_2 with long-term CPAP therapy for obstructive sleep apnea. *Am Rev Respir Dis* 135:144–147, 1987.
81. Rajagopal KR, Abbrecht PH, Tellis CJ: Control of breathing in obstructive sleep apnea. *Chest* 85:174–180, 1984.
82. Greenberg HE, Scharf SM: Depressed ventilatory load compensation in sleep apnea. Reversal by nasal CPAP. *Am Rev Respir Dis* 148:1610–1615, 1993.
83. Donahoe M, Rogers RM, Wilson DO, et al: Oxygen consumption of the respiratory muscles in normal and in malnourished patients with chronic obstructive pulmonary disease. *Am Rev Respir Dis* 140:385–391, 1989.
84. Cherniack RM: The oxygen consumption and efficiency of the respiratory muscles in health and emphysema. *J Clin Invest* 38:494–499, 1959.
85. Levison H, Cherniack RM: Ventilatory cost of exercise in chronic obstructive pulmonary disease. *J Appl Physiol* 25:21–27, 1968.
86. Fritts HW, Filler J, Fishman AP, et al: The efficiency of ventilation during voluntary hyperpnea: Studies in normal subjects and in dyspneic patients with either chronic pulmonary emphysema or obesity. *J Clin Invest* 38:1339–1348, 1959.
87. Rochester DF: Respiratory muscles and ventilatory failure: 1993 perspective. *Am J Med Sci* 305:394–402, 1993.
88. Sharp JT: The respiratory muscles in chronic obstructive pulmonary disease. *Am Rev Respir Dis* 134:1089–1091, 1986.
89. Rahn H, Otis AB, Chadwick LE, et al: The pressure-volume diagram of the thorax and lung. *Am J Physiol* 146:161–178, 1946.
90. Bellemare F, Grassino A: Effect of pressure and timing of contraction on human diaphragm fatigue. *J Appl Physiol* 53:1190–1195, 1982.
91. Fahey PJ, Hyde RW: "Won't Breath" vs "Can't Breath." Detection of depressed ventilatory drive in patients with obstructive pulmonary disease. *Chest* 84:19–25, 1983.
92. Altose MD, McCauley WC, Kelsen SG, et al: Effects of hypercapnia and inspiratory flow-resistive loading on respiratory activity in chronic airways obstruction. *J Clin Invest* 59:500–507, 1977.
93. Piper AJ, Sullivan CE: Effects of short-term NIPPV in the treatment of patients with severe obstructive sleep apnea and hypercapnia [see comments]. *Chest* 105:434–440, 1994.
94. Vincken W, Guilleminault C, Silvestri L, et al: Inspiratory muscle activity as a trigger causing the airways to open in obstructive sleep apnea. *Am Rev Respir Dis* 135:372–377, 1987.
95. Gleeson K, Zwillich CW, White DP: The influence of increasing ventilatory effort on arousal from sleep. *Am Rev Respir Dis* 142:295–300, 1990.
96. Jones JB, Wilhoit SC, Findley LJ, et al: Oxyhemoglobin saturation during sleep in subjects with and without the obesity-hypoventilation syndrome. *Chest* 88:9–15, 1985.
97. Chan CS, Grunstein RR, Bye PT, et al: Obstructive sleep apnea with se-

vere chronic airflow limitation. Comparison of hypercapnic and eucapnic patients. *Am Rev Respir Dis* 140:1274–1278, 1989.

98. Colt HG, Haas H, Rich GB: Hypoxemia vs sleep fragmentation as cause of excessive daytime sleepiness in obstructive sleep apnea. *Chest* 100:1542–1548, 1991.

99. Findley LJ, Unverzagt ME, Suratt PM: Automobile accidents involving patients with obstructive sleep apnea. *Am Rev Respir Dis* 138:337–340, 1988.

100. Guilleminault C, Connolly S, Winkle R, et al: Cyclical variation of the heart rate in sleep apnoea syndrome. Mechanisms, and usefulness of 24 h electrocardiography as a screening technique. *Lancet* 1:126–131, 1984.

101. Miller WP: Cardiac arrhythmias and conduction disturbances in the sleep apnea syndrome. Prevalence and significance. *Am J Med* 73:317–321, 1982.

102. Guilleminault C, Connolly SJ, Winkle RA: Cardiac arrhythmia and conduction disturbances during sleep in 400 patients with sleep apnea syndrome. *Am J Cardiol* 52:490–494, 1983.

103. Shepard JWJ, Garrison MW, Grither DA, et al: Relationship of ventricular ectopy to oxyhemoglobin desaturation in patients with obstructive sleep apnea. *Chest* 88:335–340, 1985.

104. Partinen M, Guilleminault C: Daytime sleepiness and vascular morbidity at seven-year follow-up in obstructive sleep apnea patients. *Chest* 97:27–32, 1990.

105. Bonsignore MR, Marrone O, Insalaco G, et al: The cardiovascular effects of obstructive sleep apneas: Analysis of pathogenic mechanisms. *Eur Respir J* 7:786–805, 1994.

106. Criteria. In: *The International Classification of Sleep Disorders Diagnostic and Coding Manual*. Rochester, American Sleep Disorders Association, 1990, pp 21–24.

107. Kribbs NB, Getsy JE, Dinges DF: Investigation and management of daytime sleepiness in sleep apnea. In: Saunders NA, Sullivan CE (eds): *Sleeping and Breathing*. New York, Marcel Dekker, 1993, pp. 575–604.

108. Walsleben JA: The measurement of daytime wakefulness. *Chest* 101:890–891, 1992.

109. Wedderburn AA: Sleeping on the job: The use of anecdotes for recording rare but serious events. *Ergonomics* 30:1229–1233, 1987.

110. Hoffstein V, Szalai JP: Predictive value of clinical features in diagnosing obstructive sleep apnea. *Sleep* 16:118–122, 1993.

111. Viner S, Szalai JP, Hoffstein V: Are history and physical examination a good screening test for sleep apnea? *Ann Intern Med* 115:356–359, 1991.

112. Kapuniai LE, Andrew DJ, Crowell DH, et al: Identifying sleep apnea from self-reports. *Sleep* 11:430–436, 1988.

113. Gyulay S, Olson LG, Hensley MJ, et al: A comparison of clinical assessment and home oximetry in the diagnosis of obstructive sleep apnea. *Am Rev Respir Dis* 147:50–53, 1993.

114. Crocker BD, Olson LG, Saunders NA, et al: Estimation of the probability of disturbed breathing during sleep before a sleep study. *Am Rev Respir Dis* 142:14–18, 1990.

115. Flemons WW, Whitelaw WA, Brant R, et al: Likelihood ratios for a sleep

apnea clinical prediction rule. *Am J Respir Crit Care Med* 150:1279–1285, 1994.

116. Sanders MH, Kern NB, Costantino JP, et al: Adequacy of prescribing positive airway pressure therapy by mask for sleep apnea on the basis of a partial-night trial. *Am Rev Respir Dis* 147:1169–1174, 1993.
117. Strollo PJ, Sanders MH, Constantino JP, et al: Split night studies for the diagnosis and treatment of sleep disordered breathing. *Sleep,* In press.
118. Krieger J: Long-term compliance with nasal continuous positive airway pressure (CPAP) in obstructive sleep apnea patients and nonapneic snorers. *Sleep* 15:S42–S46, 1992.
119. Hoffstein V, Viner S, Mateika S, et al: Treatment of obstructive sleep apnea with nasal continuous positive airway pressure. Patient compliance, perception of benefits, and side effects. *Am Rev Respir Dis* 145:841–845, 1992.
120. Practice parameters for the use of portable recording in the assessment of obstructive sleep apnea. *Sleep* 17:372–377, 1994.
121. Series F, Marc I, Cormier Y, et al: Utility of nocturnal home oximetry for case finding in patients with suspected sleep apnea hypopnea syndrome. *Ann Intern Med* 119:449–453, 1993.
122. Burrows B, Strauss RH, Niden AH: Chronic obstructive lung disease: 3. Interrelationships of pulmonary function data. *Am Rev Respir Dis* 91:861, 1965.
123. Harvey RM, Enson Y, Ferrer MI: A reconsideration of the origins of pulmonary hypertension. *Chest* 59:82, 1971.
124. Enson Y, Giuntini C, Lewis ML, et al: The influence of hydrogen ion concentration and hypoxia on the pulmonary circulation. *J Clin Invest* 43:1146, 1964.
125. Enson Y, Thomas HM, Bosken CH, et al: Pulmonary hypertension in interstitial lung disease: Relation of vascular resistance to abnormal lung structure. *Trans Assoc Am Physicians* 88:248, 1975.
126. Ungerer RG, Tahskin DP, Furst D, et al: Prevalence and clinical correlates of pulmonary arterial hypertension in progressive systemic sclerosis. *Am J Med* 75:65, 1983.
127. Guilleminault C, Dement WC: Sleep apnea syndromes and related sleep disorders. In: Williams RL, Karacan I (eds): *Sleep Disorders: Diagnosis and Treatment.* New York, Wiley, 1978.
128. Douglas NJ, Martin SE: Arousals and the sleep apnea/hypopnea syndrome. *Sleep,* In press.
129. Block AJ, Boysen PG, Wynne JW, et al: Sleep apnea, hypopnea and oxygen desaturation in normal subjects: A strong male predominance. *N Engl J Med* 300:513–517, 1979.
130. Roehrs T, Merlotti L, Petrucelli N, et al: Experimental sleep fragmentation. *Sleep* 17:438–443, 1994.
131. Stepanski E, Lamphere J, Roehrs T, et al: Experimental sleep fragmentation in normal subjects. *Int J Neurosci* 33:207–214, 1987.
132. Johns MW: A new method for measuring daytime sleepiness: The Epworth sleepiness scale. *Sleep* 14:540–545, 1991.
133. Neilly JB, Kribbs NB, Maislin G, et al: Effects of selective sleep deprivation on ventilation during recovery sleep in normal humans. *J Appl Physiol* 72:100–109, 1992.

134. Berry RB, Desa MM, Light RW: Effect of ethanol on the efficacy of nasal continuous positive airway pressure as a treatment for obstructive sleep apnea. *Chest* 99:339–343, 1991.
135. Bonora M, Shields GI, Knuth SL, et al: Selective depression by ethanol of upper airway respiratory motor activity in cats. *Am Rev Respir Dis* 130: 156–161, 1984.
136. Bonora M, St John WM, Bledsoe TA: Differential elevation by protriptyline and depression by diazepam of upper airway respiratory motor activity. *Am Rev Respir Dis* 131:41–45, 1985.
137. Leither JC, Knuth SL, Barlett D: The effect of sleep deprivation on activity of the genioglossus muscle. *Am Rev Respir Dis* 132:1242–1245, 1985.
138. Cartwright R, Ristanovic R, Diaz F, et al: A comparative study of treatments for positional sleep apnea. *Sleep* 14:546–552, 1991.
139. Strobel RJ, Rosen RC: Obesity and weight loss in obstructive sleep apnea: A critical review. *Sleep* 19:104–115, 1996.
140. Suratt PM, McTier RF, Findley LJ, et al: Effect of very-low-calorie diets with weight loss on obstructive sleep apnea. *Am J Clin Nutr* 56:182S–184S, 1992.
141. Nahmias J, Kirschner M, Karetzky MS: Weight loss and OSA and pulmonary function in obesity. *NJ Med* 90:48–53, 1993.
142. Garner D, Wooley S: Confronting the failure of behavioral and dietary treatments for obesity. *Clin Psych Rev* 11:729–780, 1991.
143. Wilson G: Behavioral treatment of obesity: Thirty years and counting. *Adv Behav Res Therapy* 16:31–75, 1994.
144. Indications and standards for use of nasal continuous positive airway pressure (CPAP) in sleep apnea syndromes. *Am J Respir Crit Care Med* 150:1738–1785, 1994.
145. Prosise GL, Berry RB: Oral-nasal continuous positive airway pressure as a treatment for obstructive sleep apnea. *Chest* 106:180–186, 1994.
146. Sanders MH, Kern NB, Stiller RA, et al: CPAP therapy via oronasal mask for obstructive sleep apnea. *Chest* 106:774–779, 1994.
147. Levinson PD, Millman RP: Causes and consequences of blood pressure alterations in obstructive sleep apnea. *Arch Intern Med* 151:455–462, 1991.
148. Kribbs NB, Pack AI, Kline LR, et al: Objective measurement of patterns of nasal CPAP use by patients with obstructive sleep apnea. *Am Rev Respir Dis* 147:887–895, 1993.
149. Reeves-Hoche MK, Hudgel DW, Meck R, et al: Continuous versus bilevel positive airway pressure for obstructive sleep apnea. *Am J Respir Crit Care Med* 151:443–449, 1995.
150. Ferguson GT, Gilmartin M: CO_2 rebreathing during BiPAP ventilatory assistance. *Am J Respir Crit Care Med* 151:1126–1135, 1995.
151. Ferguson KA, Ono T, Lowe AA, et al: A randomized crossover study of an oral appliance vs nasal-continuous positive airway pressure in the treatment of mild-moderate obstructive sleep apnea. *Chest* 109:1269–1275, 1996.
152. Schmidt-Nowara W, Lowe A, Wiegand L, et al: Oral appliances for the treatment of snoring and obstructive sleep apnea: A review. *Sleep* 18:501–510, 1995.
153. Practice parameters for the treatment of snoring and obstructive sleep apnea with oral appliances. *Sleep* 18:511–513, 1995.

154. Brownell LG, West P, Sweatman P, et al: Protriptyline in obstructive sleep apnea: A double-blind trial. *N Engl J Med* 307:1037–1042, 1982.
155. Conway WA, Zorick F, Piccione P, et al: Protriptyline in the treatment of sleep apnoea. *Thorax* 37:49–53, 1982.
156. Zwillich CW, Natalino MR, Sutton FD, et al: Effects of progesterone on chemosensitivity in normal men. *J Lab Clin Med* 92:262–269, 1978.
157. Skatrud JB, Dempsey JA, Bhansali P, et al: Ventilatory response to medroxyprogesterone acetate in normal subjects: Time course and mechanisms. *J Appl Physiol* 44:939–944, 1978.
158. Rajagopal KR, Abbrecht PH, Jabbari B: Effects of medroxyprogesterone acetate in obstructive sleep apnea. *Chest* 90:815–821, 1986.
159. Lyons HA, Huang CT: Therapeutic use of progesterone in alveolar hypoventilation associated with obesity. *Am J Med* 44:881–888, 1968.
160. Sutton FD, Zwillich CW, Creagh E, et al: Progesterone for outpatient treatment of Pickwickian syndrome. *Ann Intern Med* 83:476–479, 1975.
161. Whyte KF, Gould GA, Airlie MA, et al: Role of protriptyline and acetazolamide in the sleep apnea/hypopnea syndrome. *Sleep* 11:463–472, 1988.
162. Sharp JT, Druz WS, D'Souza V, et al: Effect of metabolic acidosis upon sleep apnea. *Chest* 87:619–624, 1985.
163. White DP, Zwillich CW, Pickett CK, et al: Central sleep apnea. Improvement with acetazolamide therapy. *Arch Intern Med* 142:1816–1819, 1982.
164. Espinoza H, Antic R, Thornton AT, et al: The effects of aminophylline on sleep and sleep-disordered breathing in patients with obstructive sleep apnea syndrome. *Am Rev Respir Dis* 136:80–84, 1987.
165. Fletcher EC, Munafo DA: Role of nocturnal oxygen therapy in obstructive sleep apnea. When should it be used? *Chest* 98:1497–1504, 1990.
166. Phillips BA, Schmitt FA, Berry DT, et al: Treatment of obstructive sleep apnea. A preliminary report comparing nasal CPAP to nasal oxygen in patients with mild OSA. *Chest* 98:325–330, 1990.
167. Chauncey JB, Aldrich MS: Preliminary findings in the treatment of obstructive sleep apnea with transtracheal oxygen. *Sleep* 13:167–174, 1990.
168. Strobel R, Lewin D, Rosen R, et al: Fenfluramine hydrochloride-assisted weight loss in obstructive sleep apnea syndrome. *Am J Respir Crit Care Med* 149:A495, 1994.
169. Stradling JR, Thomas G, Warley AR, et al: Effect of adenotonsillectomy on nocturnal hypoxaemia, sleep disturbance, and symptoms in snoring children. *Lancet* 335:249–253, 1990.
170. Aubert-Tulkens G, Hamoir M, Van dE, et al: Failure of tonsil and nose surgery in adults with long-standing severe sleep apnea syndrome. *Arch Intern Med* 149:2118–2121, 1989.
171. Shepard JWJ, Olsen KD: Uvulopalatopharyngoplasty for treatment of obstructive sleep apnea. *Mayo Clin Proc* 65:1260–1267, 1990.
172. Sher AE, Schechtman KB, Piccirillo JF: The efficacy of surgical modifications of the upper airway in adults with obstructive sleep apnea syndrome. *Sleep* 19:156–177, 1996.
173. Miljeteig H, Mateika S, Haight JS, et al: Subjective and objective assess-

ment of uvulopalatopharyngoplasty for treatment of snoring and obstructive sleep apnea. *Am J Respir Crit Care Med* 150:1286–1290, 1994.
174. Practice parameters for the use of laser-assisted uvulopalatoplasty. Standards of Practice Committee of the American Sleep Disorders Association. *Sleep* 17:744–748, 1994.
175. Riley RW, Powell NB, Guilleminault C: Obstructive sleep apnea syndrome: A review of 306 consecutively treated surgical patients. *Otolaryngol Head Neck Surg* 108:117–125, 1993.
176. Johnson NT, Chinn J: Uvulopalatopharyngoplasty and inferior sagittal mandibular osteotomy with genioglossus advancement for treatment of obstructive sleep apnea. *Chest* 105:278–283, 1994.
177. Guilleminault C, Simmons FB, Motta J, et al: Obstructive sleep apnea syndrome and tracheostomy. Long-term follow-up experience. *Arch Intern Med* 141:985–988, 1981.
178. Conway WA, Victor LD, Magilligan DJJ, et al: Adverse effects of tracheostomy for sleep apnea. *JAMA* 246:347–350, 1981.
179. Roth T, Roehrs TA, Carskadon MA, et al: Daytime sleepiness and alertness, in Kryger MH, Roth T, Dement WC. (eds): *Principles and Practice of Sleep Medicine*. Philadelphia, W.B. Saunders Company, 1994, pp.40–49.

Chapter 11

Treatment of Obesity Cardiomyopathy

Martin A. Alpert, MD
James K. Alexander, MD

Management of Congestive Heart Failure Associated with Obesity Cardiomyopathy

Diuretics, dietary salt restriction and oxygen constitute the most important immediate therapeutic measures for patients with severe congestive heart failure (CHF) associated with obesity cardiomyopathy.[1,2] Digitalis may be useful in controlling the ventricular rate in patients with atrial fibrillation and is indicated in the presence of CHF associated with left ventricular (LV) systolic dysfunction.[1,2] It is important to remember that serum digitalis levels relate to lean body mass rather than body weight.[1,3] Thus, using body weight as a guide to dosage may result in high serum digoxin levels and toxicity.[1,3] The efficacy of vasodilator therapy in obesity cardiomyopathy is uncertain. Such agents are certainly useful in the presence of systemic hypertension. Angiotensin converting enzyme inhibitors, hydralazine and nitrates, and second-generation dihydropyridine calcium channel blockers may be useful for the treatment of CHF in the presence of LV systolic dysfunction. The role of β-blockers, first-generation calcium channel blockers, and sympatholytic agents has not been defined in patients with obesity cardiomyopathy. Because thrombophlebitis and pulmonary embolism are frequently observed in patients with obesity cardiomyopathy and severe CHF, low-dose heparin prophylaxis would seem prudent.

From: Alpert MA, and Alexander JK, (eds). *The Heart and Lung in Obesity*. Armonk, NY: Futura Publishing Company, Inc., © 1998.

After effective treatment of CHF exacerbations therapy should consist of a salt-restricted (2 to 4 g of sodium per day) low calorie diet, oral diuretic therapy, oral digitalis if indicated, and oral angiotensin converting enzyme inhibitor therapy with or without additional oral vasodilator therapy if LV systolic dysfunction is present.[1,2]

Effects of Weight Loss

The most effective long-term treatment of obesity cardiomyopathy is weight loss.[1,2] Weight loss may be achieved by diet, exercise, or bariatric surgery. Both starvation and semistarvation (very low calorie) diets have been used in patients who have failed to lose weight on less restrictive diets. Surgical procedures such as jejeunoileostomy and vertical band gastroplasty have been used in individuals who have proven to be refractory to dietary therapy. Bariatric surgery is usually reserved for those who are severely obese. There is now an abundance of information concerning the effect of weight loss on cardiac morphology, central hemodynamics and LV function. Less information exists concerning the effect of weight loss on clinical cardiac manifestations in obese individuals.

Effect of Weight Loss on Cardiac Morphology, Central Hemodynamics, and LV Function

There is an increasing body of evidence to suggest that weight loss is capable of producing beneficial effects on LV morphology, central hemodynamics, and LV function in the obese. This section summarizes these changes. For a more in-depth discussion see Chapters 3, 4, 5, and 6.

Virtually all studies exploring the effects of weight loss on cardiac morphology have reported a significant decrease in mean LV mass, LV mass index, or LV mass/height index following weight loss regardless of severity of obesity prior to weight loss or the modality used to achieve weight loss.[4–8] The mechanisms by which this occurs are less clear. Some studies have reported a significant decrease in the mean LV internal dimension [4,5,8] in diastole, while others have not.[6,7] Significant decreases in mean ventricular septal and mean LV posterior wall thickness have been reported following weight loss in most studies. Similarly, the LV radius/thickness ratio has reportedly decreased significantly in some studies and not changed in others following weight loss. Studies in morbidly obese patients show that LV mass/height index decreases after weight loss primarily in patients with increased LV mass prior to weight loss.[2] Such changes relate in part to favorable alterations in LV loading conditions.[8] It is possible that such alterations may dictate morphologic changes associated with weight loss. That is, greater reduction of afterload may predispose to decreases in ventricular septal and LV posterior wall thickness, whereas greater reduction of preload may predispose to a decrease in LV cavity size.

Alaudi-din[9] reported a small, but significant decrease in mean left atrial dimension following weight loss from gastroplasty in morbidly obese patients. The effect of weight loss on right heart dimension, and epicardial fat have not been evaluated.

The effect of weight loss on central resting hemodynamics has been evaluated in moderately and severely obese patients.[9-12] These studies have consistently shown that weight loss produces significant decreases in mean oxygen consumption, mean arteriovenous oxygen difference, mean total blood volume, mean cardiac output, mean LV stroke work and mean LV work.[9-11] Mean stroke volume consistently decreased, although not always significantly.[9-11] Mean systemic vascular resistance may increase significantly with weight loss. Mean heart rate, mean pulmonary artery pressure and mean pulmonary capillary wedge pressure did not change significantly with weight loss in most studies.[9-11] The systemic blood pressure response to weight loss has been variable.[9-11]

In hypertensive obese patients, the hemodynamic response to weight loss is much the same except that blood pressure consistently decreases significantly regardless of the modality used to achieve weight loss and stroke volume and peripheral vascular resistance do not change significantly.[12-14]

Prior to weight loss the exercise-related increase in stroke volume and cardiac index is blunted, particularly in morbidly obese patients.[10, 11] After weight loss, stroke volume, (and index) and cardiac output (and index) increase to a significantly greater extent with exercise than before weight loss.[10,11]

These studies indicate that most of the adverse hemodynamic alterations associated with obesity are reversible after weight loss. Notably, limited observations suggest that LV filling pressure and pulmonary artery pressure do not change appreciably after weight loss.

Limited information is available concerning the effects of weight loss on LV diastolic filling in obese patients. In severely obese patients transmitral Doppler indices of LV diastolic filling improve after substantial weight loss from gastroplasty in those with increased LV mass.[15] These alterations are accompanied by significant decreases in

LV mass, the LV internal dimension in diastole, systolic blood pressure, and LV end-systolic wall stress.[15] Such changes are not noted in severely obese patients with normal LV mass.[15] Improvement in LV diastolic filling has also been reported following dietary weight loss.[16] Thus, it appears that improvement in LV diastolic filling following weight loss is related to regression of LV hypertrophy and favorable alterations in LV loading conditions.

The effect of weight loss on LV systolic function in the obese is variable. In one study of morbidly obese patients substantial weight loss from gastroplasty produced a significant improvement in mean LV fractional shortening in those with depressed LV fractional shortening prior to weight loss.[17] This improvement was accompanied by significant changes in the mean LV internal dimension in diastole, mean systolic blood pressure and mean LV end-systolic wall stress.[17] Such was not observed in morbidly obese patients with normal LV fractional shortening prior to weight loss.[17] In another study of severely obese patients, there was a trend toward significant improvement in LV ejection fraction after weight loss from gastroplasty despite the fact that pre-weight loss LV ejection fraction was normal.[9] In moderately obese patients weight loss from diet (but not diet plus exercise) produced a significant increase in mean LV fractional shortening in one study.[5] However, no significant change in LV systolic function was noted after weight loss in two other studies of mildly to moderately obese patients.[4,16] Notably, mean LV ejection fraction at rest decreased significantly after weight loss in hypertensive obese patients, but improved on exercise in both hypertensive and normotensive patients.[16]

LV exercise response in obese patients improves after weight loss, even in those whose LV exercise response was blunted prior to weight loss.[16]

Thus, weight loss may be accompanied by improvement in LV systolic function at rest and during exercise after weight loss in selected obese patients. Those with depressed LV systolic function prior to weight loss are most likely to experience improvement. This occurs at least in part due to favorable alterations in LV loading conditions and possibly also to regression of LV hypertrophy.

Duration of Obesity and the Effect of Weight Loss on LV Mass and Function

Patients with longer durations of obesity are more likely to experience reduction of LV mass and improvement in both diastolic and systolic LV function following weight loss.[18] Duration of obesity also correlates with the magnitude of weight loss-related alterations in the mean LV internal dimension in diastole, systolic blood pressure, and LV end-systolic wall stress.[18] Thus, those with a longer duration of obesity are more likely to experience weight loss-related regression of LV hypertrophy and improvement in LV diastolic filling and systolic function than those with a shorter duration.[18] However, it is not clear whether duration of obesity is an independent variable or appears important because of its collinear relation with LV mass and loading conditions.

Clinical Cardiac Effects of Weight Loss in Patients with Obesity Cardiomyopathy

Although the syndrome of obesity cardiomyopathy in patients with and without the sleep apnea/obesity hypoventilation syndrome has been studied extensively, relatively little information exists concerning the clinical effects of weight reduction in such individuals.

Estes and colleagues[19] reported the effects of weight loss on 6 morbidly-obese patients with the sleep apnea/obesity hypoventilation syndrome. Their ages ranged from 28 to 50 years. There were 5 men and 1 woman. All were markedly obese, and somnolent and all had periodic breathing with intermittent cyanosis. Polycythemia was present in 4, electrocardiographic right axis deviation was present in 4, and overt CHF was present in 3 patients. Weight loss ranging from 38 to 143 pounds produced reversal of these clinical manifestations in 5 of the 6 patients including all 3 with CHF.

Alpert and coworkers[20] studied 14 morbidly-obese patients with CHF before and after weight loss from gastroplasty. There were 11 women and 3 men. Ages ranged from 27 to 43 years. Mean weight decreased from 134% ± 4% overweight prior to weight loss to 40% ± 4% overweight after weight loss. New York Heart Association functional class improved from class II to class I in 5 patients; from class III to class I in 3 patients; and from class III to class II in 4 patients. New York Heart Association functional class remained unchanged in 2 class III patients. Class IV patients were not included in the study.

These studies suggest that substantial weight loss in association with appropriate medical therapy is capable of reversing many of the clinical cardiac manifestations of obesity cardiomyopathy.

Clinical Cardiac and Electrocardiographic Complications of Starvation and Semi-Starvation Diets

Case reports and small series have documented sudden death and near death in obese patients treated with a starvation diet.

In one report,[21] a 20-year-old obese woman who had lost 60 kg during therapeutic starvation with vitamin and mineral supplements experienced cardiac arrest on the seventh day of a refeeding regimen with marked QT prolongation on the post-recessitation electrocardiogram. She subsequently died of refractory ventricular fibrillation, and at necropsy paucity and gross fragmentation of cardiac myofibers was found. In another report of a 44-year-old obese diabetic woman who died with refractory lactic acidosis on a starvation regimen, biventricular hypertrophy, and scattered areas of interstitial fibrosis were noted at necropsy.[22] Two patients in a group of 12 on a therapeutic starvation regimen who died of ventricular fibrillation were found to have LV hypertrophy without other changes on postmortem examination.[23]

Severe shock without arrhythmia has also been reported in a patient on starvation regimen with vitamin and mineral supplements accompanied by marked reduction in QRS voltage and increased QT interval.[24]

The electocardiographic effect of starvation and semi-starvation diets have been examined in a number of studies.[25-37] Table 1 summarizes the results of these studies. The most common abnormality was prolongation of the corrected QT interval. Low QRS voltage and ventricular ectopy were both infrequent. Orthostatic hypotension has also been documented in the setting of severely restricted calorie dietary regimen. De Haven et al.[38] studied 7 obese subjects (6 women and 1 man, age range 23 to 38 years, weight range 120 to 169 kg) treated with a 400 kcal and isocaloric mixed diet for 5.5 weeks. Maximum mean orthostatic systolic blood pressure drop was significantly greater in the 400 kcal protein diet (-28 ± 3 mm Hg) than in the mixed diet (-18 ± 3 mm Hg). The protein diet (but not the mixed diet) also produced a 40% decline in basal plasma norepinephrine levels and a failure of plasma norepinephrine to rise after 2 minutes of standing The authors noted that compared to mixed diets, hypocaloric protein diets offer no advantage with respect to nitrogen metabolism but resulted in greater sodium depletion, a decrease in sympathetic nervous system activity and the development of orthostatic hypotension. Studies by Landsberg and Young[39] suggest the presence of central nervous system mediation of diminished sympathetic activity during dieting.

Although starvation diets with appropriate fluid, vitamin and min-

Table 1
Electrographic Effects of Starvation and Very Low Calorie Diets

Investigator	N	Gender distribution (F/M)	Age range (years)	Type of diet	Duration of diet (days)	Weight loss (kg)	Kcal	Composition of diet				
								Protein (g)	Potassium (g)	Calcium (g)	Magnesium (mg)	Copper (mg)
Pringle et al[26]	13	11/12	19–35	Starvation	53–136	20–49	0	0	0	0	0	0
Rasmussen et al[27]	22	22/0	21–53	Gastroplasty and dietary modifications	180	14–38		19–202	0.7–3.6	0.2–3.7	300	—
Langtigua et al[28]	6	5/1	21–42	VLCD; Cgn protein diet	40	13.0–14.5	300	75	1.2	0	0	0
Singer et al[29]	6	—	26–52	VLCD; 350 Kcal of meat	56–300	7–35	350	1.2/kgIBW	1.0	0.8	259	—
Linet et al[30]	14	14/0	21–41	VLCD; 350 Kcal of meat	4	—	350	1.2 kg/BW	0.4–2.3	1.2	72	—
Amatruda et al[31]	6	6/0	23–43	VLCD; Optifast (Delmark Co., Minneapolis)	40	—	472	70	2.7	1.0	49	4
Phinney et al[32]	13	13/0	21–34	VLCD	28	2.7–8.8	850	49–142	2.0	0.8–1.2	500	—
Drenik et al[33]	10	0/10	37–60	VLCD; Soy protein: 5 Cgn protein: 5	40	Soy: 19 Cgn: 20	422	Soy: 4.9 Cg: 4.7	Soy: 0.2 Cgn: 0.09	—	Soy: 123 Cgn: 23	Soy: 3.1 Cgn: 0.5
Amatruda et al[34]	5	5/0	42–58	VLCD	40	7.5–13.2	420	2.3	1.4	—	475	—

Table 1—Continued
Electrographic Effects of Starvation and Very Low Calorie Diets

Investigator	N	Gender distribution (F/M)	Age range (years)	Type of diet	Duration of diet (days)	Weight loss (kg)	Kcal	Composition of diet Protein (g)	Potassium (g)	Calcium (g)	Magnesium (mg)	Copper (mg)
Weigle et al[35]	11	0/11	49 ± 9*	VLCD; Carnation Instant Breakfast, Carnation Co, Los Angeles (plus low-fat milk)	95 ± 14*	26*	420	51	3.8	1.5	330	4
Moyer et al[36]	24	24/0	21–55	VLCD	294	11*	660–720	1.0	—	0.8	300	—
Daughtery et al[37]	12	12/0	—	VLCD; Optifast (Delmark Co., Minneapolis)	784	21*	420	70	1.96	1.0	400	2

Investigator	Comments
Pringle et al[26]	All patients were severely obese. Low voltage was noted on all electrocardiograms by week. The corrected QT interval became prolonged by week 8 in all patients and became frankly abnormal in 7. One patient suffered cardiac arrest.
Rasmussen et al[27]	Prolongation of the correct QT interval occurred within 3 months in 7 patients; no low voltage.
Langtigua et al[28]	Three subjects developed complex ventricular ectopy on Holter monitor on day 10.
Singer et al[29]	No arrhythmias or cardiovascular complications were noted.
Linet et al[30]	No electrocardiographic or cardiac complications were noted.
Amatruda et al[31]	No arrhythmias were noted on Holter monitor recordings.
Phinney et al[32]	Holter monitoring was negative in all patients and there were no changes in the corrected QT interval.
Drenik et al[33]	The corrected QT interval was prolonged at baseline in 8 and normalized during therapy.
Amatruda et al[34]	There were no changes in the QRS voltages or the corrected QT interval; 1 patient developed a 3 beat run of ventricular tachycardia.
Weigle et al[35]	There were no changes in the QRS voltage or the corrected QT interval; Holter monitoring was negative during stress testing.
Moyer et al[36]	There were no changes in QRS voltage or the corrected QT interval. One patient developed isolated ventricular premature beats during stress testing.
Daughtery et al[37]	There were no changes in the corrected QT interval. Holter monitoring was negative throughout the study.

Kcal = kilocalories; VLCD = very low calorie diet; IBW = ideal body weight; Cgn = collagen

*Average or mean values ± 1 standard deviation.

(Adapted from Fisler JS Am J Clin Nutr 56:2305–2345, 1992.)

eral supplementation have proven to be safe in most obese individuals for whom they were prescribed, there are now a sufficient number of reported instances of myocardial damage and sudden death to preclude their routine use as a safe treatment of obesity. In contrast, semistarvation or very low calorie diets with appropriate vitamin, fluid and mineral supplementation are well tolerated and appear to impart few cardiovascular complications. Bariatric surgery appears to be well tolerated from a cardiovascular standpoint.

Fisler[21] has provided an explanation for sudden cardiac deaths from severe caloric restriction that is a modification of a previous hypothesis by DeSilva.[40] This hypothesis suggests that myocardial hypertrophy from obesity predisposes to a variety of electrocardiographic abnormalities including prolongation of the QT interval. Rapid or pronounced weight loss leads to a decrease in myocardial fiber size. Lack of protein, electrolytes and micronutrients may contribute to myofibrillar damage. Such damage provides a substrate for electrical instability because of regional inhomogeneties of conduction and/or generation of abnormal impulses. Transient extracardiac stimuli, such as stress, alter sympathetic nervous system activity. Catecholamines may then act on a structurally abnormal heart to provoke life threatening arrhythmias. This hypothesis is attractive because it does not require the consistent presence of a single provoking factor to explain clinical events.

Cardiovascular Complications of Appetite Suppressant Drugs

A variety of drugs have been used to suppress appetite and aid in dietary therapy of obesity.[39] These include methamphetamine and dexedrine (both amphetamines) as well as phenylpropanolamine, phenteramine, mazindol and phendimetrazine (all amphetamine-like sympathamimetic amines).[40] All of these drugs have the capacity to stimulate heart rate and raise blood pressure. They may produce palpitations, tachycardia, and hypertension. In patients with coronary artery disease, they may produce myocardial ischemia and angina pectoris. In patients with supraventricular or ventricular ectopic beats or a history of supraventricular or ventricular tachyarrhythmias, they may produce protracted or sustained symptomatic tachyarrhythmias. They may cause worsening of hypertension in patients with established hypertension. Amphetamines may produce cardiomyopathy. For these reasons, such agents should be avoided in patients with underlying cardiovascular disease.

Newer appetite suppressant drugs (fenfluramine and dexfenflura-mine) are seratonin specific reuptake inhibitors and releasing agents.[41] Hypertension, angina pectoris, palpitations, vasodilatation, tachycar-dia, postural hypotension, peripheral vascular disease, syncope, ar-rhythmias, thrombophlebitis, pulmonary embolism, heart block, and arterial thrombosis have all been reported in patients receiving these drugs.[41] However, a cause/effect relation between these agents and the aforementioned clinical features has not been established.

The most feared complication of fenfluramine and dexfenfluramine therapy is primary pulmonary hypertension.[41,42] Primary pulmonary hypertension occurs in 1 to 2 persons per million in the general popu-lation. In those receiving fenfluramine or dexfenfluramine primary pul-monary hypertension occurs in 18 persons per million (odds ratio 9:1 in favor of primary pulmonary hypertension in such patients).[41,42] Most who have developed primary pulmonary hypertension have received the drugs longer than three months.[41,42] The mechanism by which pri-mary pulmonary hypertension occurs in such individuals is uncertain.

A recent report by Connolly et al.[43] suggests a possible relation be-tween fenfluramine and phenteramine and valvular heart disease. These authors studied 24 obese women (mean age 44 ± 8 years) who had received fenfluramine/phenteramine for 12.3 ± 7.1 months. These pa-tients had no prior heart disease and presented with cardiac murmurs and/or new cardiac symptoms. Echocardiography identified unusual valvular morphology and regurgitation in all patients, including the mi-tral and aortic valves. The affected valves had a glistening white ap-pearance and plaque-like encasement with histology similar to that noted with the carcinoid syndrome. In addition, eight patients had pul-monary hypertension with variable degrees of tricuspid regurgitation. As of the time of the report, five patients required valve surgery. In a later editorial Sobelle discusses these findings and the FDA's response.[44] The FDA has requested that reports of otherwise unexplained valvular disease or pulmonary hypertension in patients receiving fenfluramine-phenteramine be reported to the federal agency. Based on these results and anecdotal reports of valvular disease and primary pulmonary hy-pertension in patients receiving fenfluramine-phenteramine and dexfenfluramine have both been voluntarily withdrawn from the mar-ket. Sibutramine, another serotonin-specific reuptake inhibitor was re-cently approved for treatment of obesity. The only cardiovascular com-plication reported thus far with sibutramine is systemic hypertension. In considering the long-term use of pharmacotherapy for obesity, it is well to remember the conclusions of the National Task Force in the Pre-vention and Treatment of Obesity. The Task Force concluded that "pharmacotherapy for obesity, when combined with appropriate behavioral approaches to change, diet and physical activity helps some obese patients lose weight and maintain weight loss for at least one year. There is little justification for the short term use of anorexiant medications, but few studies have evaluated their safety and efficacy for more than one year. Until more data are available, pharmacotherapy cannot be recommended for routine use in obese individuals, although it may be helpful in carefully selected patients."[45] The North American Association for the Study of Obesity has recommended that a body mass index greater than 27 kg/m² be considered the minimum threshold for consideration of treatment with appetite suppressant drugs for patients without existing obesity-related comorbidities.[46]

References

1. Alexander JK: The cardiomyopathy of obesity. *Prog Cardiovasc Dis* 27: 325–334, 1985.
2. Alpert MA, Hashimi MW: Obesity and the heart. *Am J Med Sci* 3306: 117–123, 1993.
3. Ewy GA, Groves BM, Ball MF, et al: Digoxin metabolism in obesity. *Circulation* 44:810–814, 1971.
4. Himeno E, Nishino K, Nakashima Y, et al: Weight reduction regresses LV mass regardless of blood pressure level in obese subjects. *Am Heart J* 131:313–319, 1996.
5. Wirth A, Kröger H: Improvement in LV morphology and function in obese subjects following a diet and exercise program. *Int J Obes* 19:61–66, 1995.
6. MacMahon SW, Wilcken DEL, MacDonald CJ: The effect of weight reduction on LV mass. A randomized controlled trial in young, overweight hypertensive patients. *N Engl J Med* 314:334–339, 1986.
7. Jordan J, Messerli FH, Lavie CJ, et al: Reduction of weight and LV mass with serotonin uptake inhibition in obese patients with systemic hypertension. *Am J Cardiol* 75:743–744, 1995.
8. Alpert MA, Lambert CR, Terry BE, et al: Effect of weight loss on LV mass in non-hypertensive morbidly obese patients. *Am J Cardiol* 73.918–921, 1994.
9. Alaud-din A, Meterissian S, Lisbona R, et al: Assessment of cardiac function in patients who are morbidly obese. *Surgery* 108:809–820, 1990.
10. Alexander JK, Peterson KL: Cardiovascular effects of weight reduction. *Circulation* 45:310–318, 1972.
11. Backman L. Freyschuss U, Hallberg D, et al: Reversibility of cardiovascular changes in extreme obesity. Effects of weight reduction through jejeunoileostomy. *Acta Med Scand* 205:367–373, 1979.
12. Reisen E, Frohlich ED, Messerli FH, et al: Cardiovascular changes after weight reduction in obesity hypertension. *Ann Intern Med* 98:315–319, 1983.

13. Foely EF, Benotti PN, Borlane BL, et al: Impact of gastric restrictive surgery on hypertension in the morbidly obese. *Am J Surg* 163:294–297, 1992.

14. Carson JL, Ruddy ME, Duff AE, et al: The effect of gastric bypass surgery on hypertension in the morbidly obese. *Arch Intern Med* 154:193–200, 1994.

15. Alpert MA, Lambert CR, Terry BE, et al: Effect of weight loss on LV diastolic filling in morbid obesity. *Am J Cardiol* 76:1198–1201, 1995.

16. DasGupta P, Rasmhanmdany E, Brigden G, et al: Improvement in LV function after rapid weight loss in obesity. *Eur Heart J* 13:1060–1066, 1992.

17. Alpert MA, Terry BE, Lambert CR, et al: Factors influencing LV systolic function in non-hypertensive morbidly obese patients, and effect of weight loss induced by gastroplasty. *Am J Cardiol* 71:733–737, 1993.

18. Alpert MA, Lambert CR, Panayiotou H, et al: Relationship of duration of morbid obesity to LV mass, systolic function and diastolic filling and effect of weight loss. *Am J Cardiol* 76:1194–1197, 1995.

19. Estes EH, Sieker HO, McIntosh HD, et al: Reversible cardiopulmonary syndrome with extreme obesity. *Circulation* 41:179–187, 1957.

20. Alpert MA, Terry BE, Mulekar M, et al: Cardiac morphology and LV function in morbidly obese patients with and without congestive heart failure, and effect of weight loss. *Am J Cardiol* 80:736–740, 1997.

21. Garnett ES, Barnard DL, Ford J, et al: Gross fragmentation of cardiac myofibrils after therapeutic starvation for obesity. *Lancet* 1:914–916, 1963.

22. Cubberly PT, Polsher SA, Schulman CL: Lactic acidosis and death after the treatment of obesity by fasting. *N Engl J Med* 272:628–630, 1965.

23. Spencer IOB: Death during therapeutic starvation for obesity. *Lancet* 1:1288–1289, 1968.

24. Sandhofer F, Dienste F, Botszanco K, et al: Severe cardiovascular complication associated with prolonged starvation. *Br Med J* 1:462–463, 1973.

25. Fisler JS: Cardiac effects of starvation and semistarvation diets: Safety and mechanisms of actions. *Am J Clin Nutr* 56:2305–2345, 1992.

26. Pringle TH, Scobie TH, Marrage RG, et al: Prolongation of the QT interval during therapeutic styarvation: A substrate for malignant arrhythmias. *Int J Obes* 7:253–261, 1983.

27. Rasmussen LH, Anderson T: The relationship between QTc changes and nutrition during weight loss after gastroplasty. *Acta Med Scand* 217:271–275, 1985.

28. Lantigua RA, Amatruda JM, Biddle TL, et al: Cardiac arrhythmias associated with a liquid protein diet for treatment of obesity. *N Engl J Med* 303:735–738, 1980.

29. Singer DL: Twenty-four hour Holter monitoring facts to diagnose significant cardiac arrhythmias in six patients on prolonged protein sparing fast. *Obes Metab* 1:159–164, 1981.

30. Linet OI, Butler D, Caswel K, et al: Absence of cardiac arrhythmias during a very low calorie diet with high biological quality protein. *Int J Obes* 7:313–320, 1983.

31. Amatruda OM, Biddle TL, Patten ML, et al: Vigorous supplementation of a hypocaloric diet prevents cardiac arrhythmias and mineral depletion. *Am J Med* 74:1016–1022, 1983.

32. Phinney SD, Bistriar BP, Kosiwski E, et al: Normal cardiac rhythm during hypocaloric diets of varying carbohydrate content. *Arch Intern Med* 148:873–877, 1983.
33. Drenick EJ, Blumfield DE, Fisler JS, et al: Cardiac function during very low calorie reducing diet with dietary protein of good and poor nutritional quality. In: Blackburn GL, Bray GA (eds): *Management of Obesity by Severe Caloric Restriction.* Littleton, MA: DSG Publishing, 1985, pp 223–234.
34. Amatruda OM, Richeson OF, Welle SC, et al: The safety and efficacy of a controlled low energy ("very low calorie") diet in the treatment of non-insulin-dependent diabetes and obesity. *Arch Intern Med* 148:873–877, 1988.
35. Weigle DS, Callahan DB, Fellows CL, et al: Preliminary assessment of very low calorie diets by conventional and signal-averaged electrocardiography. *Int J Obes* 13:691–677, 1989.
36. Moyer CL, Hilly RG, Amsterdam EA, et al: Effects of cardiac stress during a very low calorie diet and exercise program in obese women. *Am J Clin Nutr* 53:854–858, 1989.
37. Doherty JU, Wadden TA, Zuke L, et al: Long-term evaluation of cardiac function in obese patients treated with a very-low caloric diet: A controlled clinical study of proteins without underlying heart disease. *Am J Clin Nutr* 53:854–858, 1991.
38. DeHaven J, Sherwin R, Hendler R, et al: Nitrogen and sodium balance and sympathetic nervous system activity in obese subjects treated with a low-calorie protein or mixed diet. *N Engl J Med* 302:477–482, 1980.
39. Landsberg LS, Young JB: Fasting, feeding and regulation of the sympathetic nervous system. *N Engl J Med* 298:1295–1301, 1978.
40. DeSilva RA: Ionic catecholamine and dietary effects of cardiac rhythm. In: Blackburn GL, Bray GA (eds), *Management of Obesity by Severe Caloric Restriction.* Littleton MA: PSG Publishing, 1985, pp 183–204.
41. *Physicians Desk Reference,* Montvale NJ, Medical Economics Co., 1997, pp 1035, 786, 422, 2648, 2662, 1615, 2239, 687, 2911 and 2423.
42. Abenhaim L, Moride Y, Brenot F, et al: Appetite suppressant drugs and the risk of primary pulmonary hypertension. *N Engl J Med* 335:609–619, 1996.
43. Connolly HM, Crasy JL, McGoon MD, et al: Valvular heart disease associated with fenfluramine—phentramine. *N Engl J Med* 337:581–588, 1997.
44. Sobelle R: Fen-phen and risk of valvular disease. *Circulation* 196:1705–1706, 1997.
45. National Task Force on the Prevention and Treatment of Obesity. Long-term pharmacotherapy in the management of obesity. *JAMA* 276:1907–1915, 1996.
46. Guidelines for the approval and use of drugs to treat obesity: A position paper of the North American Association for the Study of Obesity. *Obes Res* 3:473–478. 1995.

Chapter 12

Obesity and
Coronary Heart Disease

James K. Alexander, MD

Prevalence of Obesity

The prevalence of obesity in the United States is significant and increasing. Using cutoff points for obesity as body mass index (BMI, weight/height²) over 27.8 kg/m² for men and 27.3 kg/m² for women (approximately 124% and 120% of desirable weight, respectively[1]) the prevalence of obesity in the National Health and Nutrition Examination Survey (NHANES) increased during the period between 1976 and 1980 (NHANES II), from 25.4% to 33.3% during the period between 1988 and 1991 (NHANES III) in subjects 20 to 74 years of age.[2] These overall figures are similar to those for Caucasian men, Caucasian women, and African-American men, but percentages for African-American women were 43.1 and 49.2, respectively. The prevalence of childhood obesity is also significant. According to recent estimates, 27.1% of 6 to 11 year olds, and 21.9% of 12 to 18 year olds are obese, with a higher incidence in girls (25.5% vs. boys 18.3%)[3] This has implications from a preventional standpoint, because about 70% of pre-adolescent obese children remain obese as adults.[4]

Methodology and Data Analysis

Several approaches to the relation of obesity to coronary heart disease (CHD) have evolved: (1) epidemiological studies relating CHD

From: Alpert MA, and Alexander JK, (eds). *The Heart and Lung in Obesity.* Armonk, NY: Futura Publishing Company, Inc., © 1998.

morbidity and/or mortality to some measure of total body fat, or visceral adiposity; (2) cross-sectional studies examining the relation of body fat to coronary anatomic disease; (3) correlation of the incidence of coronary risk factors with various measures of adiposity; and (4) epidemiological studies designed to prove or disprove a unique causal atherogenic mechanism (obesity as an independent risk factor) relating to obesity.

Obesity is not homogeneous, and fat patterning varies with gender, age, ethnicity, and heredity. Four obesity phenotypes have been identified based on anatomic fat distribution[5:] (1) excess total fat mass; (2) excess subcutaneous truncal-abdominal fat; (3) excess abdominal visceral fat; and (4) excess gluteal-femoral fat.

The distinction between obesity and overweight is important. Because accurate measures of body fat have significant limitations in terms of cost, convenience, simplicity, or logistical considerations, relative weight, BMI, skinfold thicknesses, and waist/hip circumference ratio (WHR) have commonly been taken as surrogate measures of body fat in large scale epidemiological studies. Relative weight does not accurately reflect adiposity. Using computed tomography as the reference standard, weight for height indices such as BMI predict total adipose tissue mass with an error of about 10%.[6] However, the relation between BMI and fatness is not the same in women as in men, and is not the same for all ages.[7] Skinfold measurements may be used to estimate volume of subcutaneous fat, but are inexact for visceral fat mass, even though correlated to some extent with radiographic measurements.[8] Formulae for skinfold measurements at three body sites correlating with total fat mass as estimated by body density have been developed, but a prediction error of 40% or more may be expected in obese subjects.[9] Furthermore, difficulty in identifying anatomic sites and other factors reduce the accuracy of skinfold regression equations in very obese subjects.[9] Indices such as WHR predict visceral adipose tissue volume with an error of at least 15% to 20% as compared with computed tomographic estimates.[6] Despite its epidemiological value, WHR has at least two drawbacks. The ratio is difficult to interpret biologically and changes in body fat or visceral fat may produce little change in the ratio.[10] Thus, anthropometric measurements suitable for epidemiological studies leave a significant margin of error in the appraisal of the obese state, with considerable potential for misclassification. In an effort to determine whether obesity per se is an independent risk factor for the development or progression of CHD, multivariate analysis has been carried out to control for recognized CHD risk factors. Difficulties in the interpretation of such studies stem from the potential impact of the interactions between weight and diet, physical activity, coronary risk factors, and other conditions.[11] Thus a major difficulty with interpretation of these studies revolves around the attempt to relate a single entity, which is itself conditioned by a variety of factors, to another complex interaction of factors conditioning CHD mortality and morbidity. These interactions are not easily characterized by mathematical models, and the question of whether those predictions for nonobese subjects are equally valid for obese subjects has received little attention.

Obesity, CHD Mortality and Morbidity

Reviews of epidemiological studies examining the relation of obesity to CHD mortality and morbidity have emphasized the pattern of conflicting results.[12, 13] Manson et al.[14] and Sjostrum[15] note that failure to control for smoking, failure to eliminate early mortality due to pre-existing disease, and inappropriate control for intermediate risk factors (hypertension, dyslipidemia, diabetes) by which obesity may exert adverse effects, are frequent shortcomings in these studies, leading to questionable results. In addition, Sjostrum[15] cites misclassification bias, small cohort size and/or short-term follow-up, and dilution of the statistical effect of high-risk subgroups when all obese are surveyed, as factors minimizing a positive relation. Sjootrum[15] found that in studies longer than 6 years with cohort populations of greater than 20,000 participants there was a positive relation between obesity and overall mortality. However, several smaller studies involving 1000 to 2000 men aged 40 to 65 years followed for 10 to 15 years have indicated that obesity has predictive power for CHD mortality when relative weight is greater than 140% of "desirable" or BMI is greater than 30 kg/m^2.[16–21]

Some studies are noteworthy in that cohort size is relatively large, follow up is relatively long, and the focus is on CHD mortality. The relation between BMI and risk ratio for CHD mortality as reported in these studies is depicted in Figure 1 men, and in Figure 2 for women. With the exception of the Nurses' Health Study[24] (n = 115,195), these were general population studies of large scale, all with follow-up periods ranging from 10 to 16 years. There was no control for smoking except in the studies of Seidell et al,[23] Manson et al,[24] and Rissanen et al[27] where the data selected are from the nonsmoking cohorts. It appears that men with a BMI of greater than 30 kg/m^2 and women with a BMI of greater than 27 are at increased risk. The data depicted in these graphs encompass an age range of 25 to 69 years. The relation between

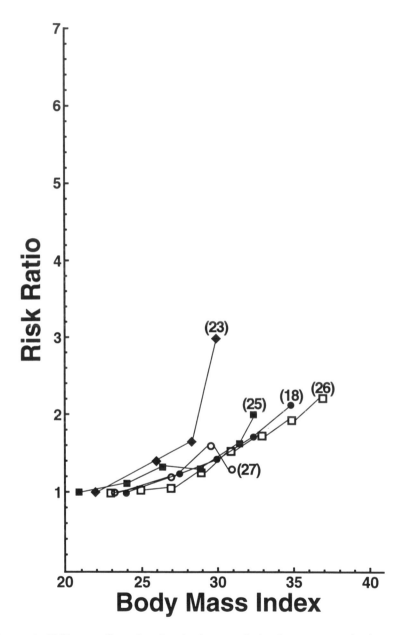

Figure 1. CHD mortality related to body mass index in men over the long term. Numbers refer to reference cited.

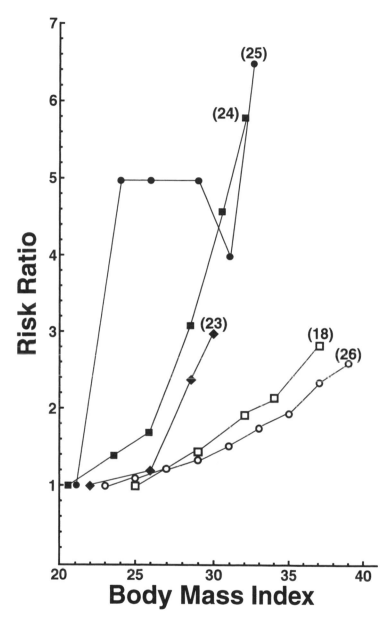

Figure 2. CHD mortality related to body mass index in women over the long term. Numbers refer to reference cited.

BMI and CHD mortality is considerably less pronounced in the age range 70 to 89 years.[22, 27] Because these studies demonstrate a positive relation between BMI and CHD mortality, in some cases with short-comings as noted above, it may be argued that the relation might have been stronger had the study design been less vulnerable.[15] Thus, it seems reasonable to conclude that total fat mass, or at least obesity as appraised in epidemiological studies, influences CHD mortality in some general populations. Perhaps of equal or greater importance from a public health standpoint is the increased CHD mortality observed in overweight adolescents (13 to 18 years) who participated in the Harvard Growth Study,[28] with 13-year follow-up.

Nevertheless, it is appropriate to recognize that a significant positive relation between BMI or overweight and CHD has not been found in all settings. Analysis of male cohorts in the Pooling Project indicates no clear age adjusted or age specific association of obesity with CHD or CHD mortality.[12] In the Twin Cities Prospective Study, 284 "healthy" male executives aged 45 to 55 years were followed for 35 years. Body fat, as assessed by BMI, skinfold thickness, relative girth, and body density, did not significantly discriminate the 35 year dead from survivors.[29] In the Charleston Heart Study, neither BMI nor fat patterning predicted CHD mortality during 25 to 28 years of follow-up in African-American women.[30] Mexican Americans, a population with a high incidence of obesity, have the same mortality rate as non-Hispanic white Americans, which suggests that obesity does not increase their death rate.[31] These and other data indicate that obesity and excess total fat mass may have little affect on CHD mortality in selected sex, ethnic, social, and racial groups, and that other factors such as physical activity may impact on CHD mortality to a greater extent than total fat mass or obesity. Meta-analysis indicates that physical activity has a favorable impact on the risk of CHD and CHD death with or without covariate adjustment for overweight.[31] Thus increased physical activity of overweight subjects may blunt the potential adverse effects of obesity. In the United States, the CHD mortality rate has decreased since the 1970s despite an increase in the population percentage of overweight subjects.[32]

Anatomic Studies: Obesity and CHD

A number of cross-sectional studies examining a possible correlation between the anatomic extent of CHD and indices of obesity at necropsy have been carried out. In an autopsy series of military personnel, Yater and colleagues[33] found no difference between the weights of 233 men who died of coronary disease versus the weights of all inductees in the same age group and/or the weights of 297 men who died accidentally. Lee and Thomas[34] found no differences between weights of 450 persons aged 30 to 60 years who died of acute myocardial infarction and average weights for the general population matched for age and sex. In an autopsy series of 408 subjects aged 15 to 89 years, programmed to examine the extent of coronary atheroma, no difference was found among underweight, normal, and overweight persons.[35] In a meticulous study of 110 autopsied subjects in whom subcutaneous fat tissue biopsies were examined, Bjurulf[36] found that the severity of coronary atherosclerosis correlated with the size of fat cells, but not with the number. This was interpreted as an indication of a predominance of environmental versus genetic factors in the pathogenesis of CHD. In a retrospective study, Ackerman and colleagues[37] found the degree of coronary sclerosis the same in persons of average weight versus overweight persons at autopsy. Using BMI as an obesity index, Wilkens and colleagues[38] found evidence for greater severity of CHD and incidence of catastrophic coronary events in obese nonhypertensive men, but not in women. In an autopsy series of 137 Japanese-American men there was some correlation between severity of CHD and relative weight greater than 116%.[39] With the exception of Yater's study, which included accidental deaths, the interpretation of these necropsy data is subject to the reservation that the nutritional status of the individual at postmortem examination may not reflect that which existed during the development of the atheromatous lesions. However, the observations by Montenegro and Salberg[40] at autopsy that included accidental deaths obviate this limitation. This is a report of the International Atherosclerosis Project 1960 to 1964 involving autopsy data in 350 persons from 6 different geographic and ethnic populations. In 350 subjects the relation between fatty streaks or raised atheromatous lesions and body weight, trunk length, and thickness of subcutaneous fat was meticulously catalogued. The authors found that those who died of CHD were slightly more obese than those who died of natural causes, but concluded that this was due to inclusion of wasting diseases. For those whose death was accidental, there was no association between the extent of coronary atheroma and any of the indices of overweight or obesity in the population as a whole or in any of the individual groups. In another World Health Organization international study in Europe,[41] a standardized average atherosclerosis group was used to exclude the effects of wasting disease. Neither the prevalence of coronary stenosis nor the extent of atherosclerotic lesions were increased for the group of obese as compared with thin subjects when hypertensives and diabetics were excluded. In a review of autopsy studies in 1983, these same conclusions were reached.[42] However, autopsy studies focusing on findings under circumstances of accidental death utilizing somewhat more precise measures of adiposity and quantitating the severity of coronary atheromatous involvement more accurately, have demonstrated some correlations of CHD with obesity. In a study of 672 autopsy cases of men aged 25 to 64 years, about 70% of which followed accidental death, there was a weak association ($P = .073$) between abdominal panniculus thickness and raised coronary artery lesions in Causcasian men, but not African-Americans.[43] Autopsy examinations of a larger group of men (1108) aged 25 to 44 years who died of causes other than CHD or CHD-related disease, uncontrolled for smoking, demonstrated a correlation between body weight-height indices and coronary raised lesions (RLCA), and between panniculus thickness and RLCA in Caucasians but not African-Americans.[44] However, there were only slight differences in obesity indices between this group and those who died of CHD. A recent multicenter study has quantified aortic and right coronary atherosclerosis in 1532 young persons who died of external causes in relation to BMI and thickness of the panniculus adiposus.[45] Percentages of fatty streaks and raised lesions in the right coronary artery were significantly increased in men aged 25 to 34 years with BMI greater than 30, and these values were 2 to 4 times higher with panniculus thickness greater than 17 mm, suggesting an additional effect of central obesity. It is noteworthy, however, that no relation to adiposity was found in women. An attempt to establish obesity as an independent risk factor in men is blunted by limitation of case number and sources of error in lipid plasma measurements, and lack of information about blood pressure. Nevertheless, the findings establish a relation between obesity and the anatomic extent of coronary disease with BMI >30 in men, consonant with the implications of epidemiological studies. It is interesting that the conclusion is not greatly different from that drawn by Wilens in 1947.[46] In a comparison of severity of coronary atherosclerosis in 1260 autopsied cases, with gradations of poor, average, or obese nutritional status, and that used an abdominal panniculus of 3 cm or more (which is quite large) as evidence of obesity, Wilens[46] found that advanced atherosclerosis occurred twice as often with obesity as with poor nutritional status in all age groups. If greater degrees of obesity were associated with greater predisposition to CHD, severe obesity might be expected to carry the greatest risk. However, postmortem studies on extremely obese subjects over an age range of 30 to 75 years reveal little or no coronary atheromatous disease.[47–49] Of 1320 young men with BMI ≥31 kg/m^2 examined for military service in Denmark during the periods between 1943 to 1973 and 1964 to 1973, 19 died before July 1974; only 2 were due to myocardial infarction.

A number of cross-sectional studies have been performed that examined the relation between indices of obesity and severity of coronary disease as indicated arteriographically. All 12 of the studies reviewed here showed no correlation of coronary disease severity with BMI or other weight-height index.[51–62] In a study of 262 patients with established CHD, repeat coronary arteriography 2 to 182 months later demonstrated no difference in progression of disease in those with relative weight greater than 120% vs. those with lesser relative weight.[53] In the Honolulu Heart Program, 357 men of a cohort of 7591 free of CHD at entry had arteriographic studies during a 20-year follow-up period. Taking the 35 men with less than 50% stenosis of one artery as controls, BMI did not separate controls from those with greater degrees of stenosis in the total arteriography series, nor in the arteriography series of total minus infarction.[57] Thus, neither cross-sectional nor longitudinal arteriographic studies have demonstrated any clear relation between total fat mass and extent of coronary atheromatous disease. In contrast, while showing no relation to BMI, a positive correlation between WHR or visceral abdominal adipose tissue mass and severity of coronary disease has been found in several studies.[55,58,60–62] However, the association has not been uniform. In one study there was a negative correlation.[59] In another, a positive correlation emerged in older women, but not in men or younger women.[55] Two studies demonstrated a correlation only after allowing for established risk factors.[60,61]

Thus, epidemiological studies indicate an association of CHD mortality and a certain level of obesity or total fat mass, while with rare exception, anatomic studies have demonstrated no or marginal correlation with presence or severity of disease. This disparity has at least two important implications relative to obesity and CHD. First, failure to find a reasonably consistent association in the anatomic studies provides evidence that total fat mass by itself has little or no impact on the coronary atheromatous process. Second, epidemiological evidence is based on clinical events, whereas anatomic information relates to severity of atheroma deposition and coronary stenosis. It is well recognized that the incidence of myocardial infarction and unstable angina, the harbingers of CHD mortality and morbidity, does not correlate well with the severity of atheromatous stenosis, which characteristically develops at sites of plaque ulceration or rupture with clot formation and complete or partial coronary occlusion.[63,64] While the precise mechanisms leading to instability of atheratomatous lesions are still under investigation, the process appears to be initiated by endothelial dysfunction and injury, related to shear stress, hypertension, dyslipidemia, and diabetes.[64] Thus, epidemiological but not anatomic studies reflect coronary mortality and morbidity mediated through the development of risk factor mechanisms associated with excess total fat mass. The extent to which excess visceral abdominal fat is associated with accelerated progression of CHD has not been clearly defined, although the weight of evidence suggests a positive, though not clearly independent, impact.

Regional Fat Distribution

Some epidemiological studies that use WHR or subscapular skin fold thickness as indices of abdominal visceral (mesenteric and omental) fat have identified central adiposity as a condition associated with increased CHD morbidity and mortality independent of total body fat mass.[24, 65–72] Whereas there is a J-shaped association or no correlation at all between BMI and CHD in these studies, increasing WHR tends to correlate monotomically with CHD risk. In these subjects, particularly in women, there tends to be a clustering of coronary risk factors, including dyslipoproteinemia, and noninsulin-dependent diabetes mellitus (NIDDM), as well as hypertension and hyperandrogenisin[69,73,74] In men the incidence of these risk factors increases steeply when the WHR is greater than 1.0, and in women when it is >0.8. However, WHR cutoff points, which are largely based primarily on data from Caucasian populations, may not be appropriate for women, older individuals, or some racial groups in the United States.[75] The pathogenetic basis for some of these factors appears to be related to unique metabolic characteristics of intra-abdominal as compared to other adipose tissue. Because of a preponderance of β-adrenergic receptors, portal tissue has a very sensitive system for mobilization of free-fatty acids (FFA). A high flux of FFA to the liver through the portal circulation stimulates hepatic triglyceride production, very low density lipoprotein secretion, and reduces hepatic extraction of insulin, leading to hyperinsulinemia and insulin resistance (Figure 3).[76,77]

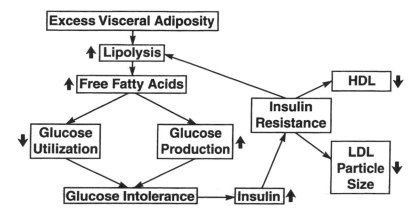

Figure 3. Metabolic alterations associated with visceral abdominal adiposity. Schema based on data presented in Reference 159.

Obesity and CHD Risk Factors

Of the established CHD risk factors encountered with increased frequency in obese subjects, those discussed here include dysipidemia, diabetes, hypertension, and hyperuricemia.

Plasma low-density lipoprotein cholesterol (LDL) and high-density lipoprotein (HDL) levels are highly associated with CHD incidence.[78] With increasing BMI, levels of LDL and triglycerides tend to rise progressively while HDL levels fall.[79] Total cholesterol levels correlate less well or not at all with BMI,[68,79-81] especially in older subjects. However, in very obese women (BMI >35 kg/m²) with normal glucose tolerance there is no linear relation to these parameters, which appears to reach a threshold at a BMI of approximately 30.[82] Correlations between central obesity, as indicated by WHR, and these atherogenic lipid alterations are higher and more consistent.[68,81,83,84] In addition, central obesity is associated with a preponderance of the small dense LDL fraction, and increased concentrations of small very low-density lipoprotein (VLDL),[83] a metabolic disorder recognized as a CHD risk factor.[85] Diabetes has been consistently associated with CHD in epidemiological studies.[78, 86] The association of overweight with NIDDM is well established,[87,88] and tends to increase with increasing BMI.[81] However, body fat distribution is of greater importance than BMI in relation to glucose and insulin metabolism.[68,72,84,89] In association with increased pancreatic secretion and diminished hepatic uptake of insulin, hyperinsulinemia, insulin resistance, and NIDDM commonly accompany abdominal obesity.[84,90] Analysis of the epidemiological data does not support the notion that hyperinsulinemia is an independent major risk factor for CHD.[91] A distinction must be made, however, between hyperinsulinemia and insulin resistance. Although insulin resistance has been proposed as an independent risk factor for CHD,[92] it has been linked to increased triglyceride and reduced HDL levels.[93] Glucose intolerance, plasma insulin levels, and truncal fat are inversely correlated with plasma HDL levels, but not with total body fat.[94] The association with CHD does not imply that insulin resistance itself is atherogenic,[95] and it has been suggested that it is a marker of other hormonal, metabolic, and neuroendocrine abnormalities not adequately assessed by studying conventional risk factors.[96] In support of the thesis of a strong genetic component in central obesity and its metabolic linkages, apoprotein-D (Apo-D) genotype differences have been found between obese subjects and slim controls, and associations between Apo-D gene polymorphism and both fasting insulin and NIDDM in the obese.[97] Since several genes involved in the regulation of lipoprotein-lipid levels have been reported to show polymorphism, abdominal visceral obesity may be considered as a permissive factor that exacerbates susceptibility to dyslipidemia rather than a primary regulation of the dyslipidemic state.[98] That genetic factors may also play a role in the association of excess total fat mass with an atherogenic lipid profile is suggested by the relation of Clara cell protein 1 (P1), secreted by bronuchiolar epithelial cells, to dyslipidemia. Clara cell P1 serum levels increase as a function of BMI, and correlate positively with LDL levels, and negatively with HDL levels.[99]

Large-scale population studies indicate that the prevalence of hypertension in overweight individuals is clearly higher than that in subjects of normal weight. In the Nationwide Community Hypertension Evaluation Clinic screening program of more than 1 million people, relative frequency of hypertension in overweight as compared with normal weight screens ranged from 1.98 to 2.69 for ages 20 to 39 years, and from 1.31 to 1.59 for ages 40 to 64 years.[100] Correlation of relative weight and BMI with blood pressure levels is higher in children,[101] young adults,[102] and women[103] than in men, falling at middle age.[102] Development of hypertension may accompany weight gain with advanced age.[104] However, the majority of obese youngsters are not hypertensive, and some of the most obese are normotensive.[105] Even one-third of extremely obese adults are normotensive.[106] Although the risk of hypertension is increased with overweight, the correlation of hypertension with overweight is of a low order,[107,108] indicating that most of hypertension is not obesity induced.

Of particular interest from a public health standpoint is the significant overrepresentation of CHD risk factors in children and adolescents aged 5 to 18 years with percent body fat levels (estimated from skinfold measurements) above 25% in males and above 30% in females.[109] A secular trend toward increasing obesity in this group has been observed over the last 15 years in the Bogalusa Heart Study.[110] This secular trend has been accomoanied by increasing CHD risk.[111] Longitudinal studies indicate that overweight children and adolescents tend to become overweight adults.[112–114] For a review of obesity and CHD risk factors in youth, see Gidding et al.[115]

Gout has been found to be positively related to CHD mortality in women aged 55 to 64 years, and was adjudged to be an important CHD risk factor for postmenopausal women in the Chicago Heart Association Detection Project in Industry.[116] The well-known association of gout with more severe degrees of obesity may well be a contributing factor to CHD mortality of obese subjects that has received little attention in epidemiological studies. Other CHD risk factors significantly increased with NIDDM and central adiposity include whole blood and plasma viscosity, and fibrinogen levels.[117] Failure to account for the ever increasing number of CHD risk factors and their relation to obesity in epidemiological studies has biased some toward unjustified interpretations suggesting excess total or abdominal fat mass as independent CHD risk factors.

Obesity as an Independent Risk Factor for CHD

Use of the term independent risk factor would imply the existence of a mechanism unique to the factor in question that impacts positively on the development or progression of the atheromatous process, or on its clinical manifestations. In practice, from an epidemiological standpoint, this term has been used to record a component of incidence risk that remains unaccounted for when established risk factors are entered into multivariate analysis of the data. Thus, in some sense as applied to obesity, it represents an association by default. Meta-analysis of epidemiological studies of CHD risk factors in which obesity was included as a putative factor have generally indicated its absence as appraised by relative weight or height-weight indices.[12, 118] A notable exception is the Framingham Study.[119] However, as noted by Keys [29] on re-analysis of the data, CHD mortality was not significantly related to body weight, and failure to consider other obesity-related risk factors (vide supra) was suggested by Sjostrum[15] as accounting for the result. The absence of a reasonably consistent correlation between total or peripheral fat mass and severity of atheromatous disease as appraised at autopsy or on arteriography further emphasizes the disparity between overall fatness per se and CHD. Obesity per se, as indicated by relative weight or weight-height indices, has not been listed as a coronary risk factor for CHD in the National Cholesterol Education Program reports.[120] Excess visceral abdominal fat, however, has been considered to be an independent risk factor for CHD.[70] Diabetes, hypertriglyceridemia, reduced fibrinolysis, hyperinsulinemia, and insulin resistance may be linked to elevated portal vein FFA concentrations secondary to increased visceral abdominal fat.[121,122] Nevertheless, this metabolic profile may be found in some normal weight individuals with large abdominal fat mass, and not all viscerally obese subjects are at high risk for CHD. Genetic sensitivity to diabetes and dyslipidemia appear to be exacerbated by visceral adiposity, thus accounting for the heterogeneous outcome.[123]

Thus, the evidence at this time indicates that the effect of excess total body fat on CHD is mediated through enhancement of atherogenic factors that leads to progression of disease, and the effect of excess total or abdominal visceral fat in this regard may be greater in genetically susceptible individuals.

Weight Loss in Obese Subjects

A meta-analysis of effects of dieting on blood lipids and lipoproteins indicates that weight reduction is associated with significant decreases and correlations for total cholesterol (TC), LDL, VLDL, and triglyceride levels.[124] For every kilogram decrease in body weight, a 0.009 mmol/L increase in HDL occurred for subjects at a stabilized reduced weight. Decrease in VLDL levels with weight loss comes about as a result of decreased production secondary to reduced FFA flux and hyperinsulinemia, and increased clearance due to enhanced lipoprotein lipase activity.[69,125] Decrements in triglyceride and increments in HDL plasma levels appear to be more consistent than changes in TG or LDL with weight reduction.[126] Studies of very obese subjects before and after gastric bypass or stapling procedures have demonstrated significant changes in lipid levels, generally affecting HDL and triglycerides to a greater extent than LDL,[127–131] although LDL size increased in one study.[131] Although favorable alterations of lipid levels may accompany a dietary regimen for weight loss with or without exercise,[132] HDL levels may increase more in those who exercise, at least in men.[133] A greater tendency to normalization of lipid levels with weight loss in adolescents takes place in those with abdominal obesity than in those with gluteal-femoral obesity.[134] However, weight reduction by diet and exercise of about 6 kg in moderately obese older women is not sufficient to modify lipid levels.[135]

In obese subjects with glucose intolerance and hyperinsulinemia, substantial weight reduction is usually accompanied by improvement in these parameters.[136, 137] This effect is brought about by enhanced glucose oxidation and improved insulin sensitivity.[138] In subjects with either increased total or abdominal fat mass, weight loss results in a fall in fasting plasma insulin levels associated with increased insulin sensitivity.[134,139]

Sustained weight reduction results in lowering of blood pressure in 50% or more of hypertensive overweight subjects, often to normal levels.[108,140–142] Blood pressure reduction with weight loss is independent of age and degree of obesity, usually occurring early with modest decrements of 5% to 10% in weight,[143,144] reaching a plateau over a period of several months with continued weight loss.[145] Average fall in blood pressure per kilogram weight loss over a period of months has been found to be 1 to 4 mm Hg systolic and 1 to 2 mm Hg diastolic, with considerable variability.[146] Salt restriction tends to augment blood pressure reduction with weight loss, but the decremental effect is independent of salt,[147,148] and energy restriction.[149] For reviews, see Weinsier et al.[18] and Seidell et al.[23]

Uric acid serum levels tend to fall with weight loss, but the degree of obesity has little influence on the magnitude of change, nor is there any significant correlation between decrements in weight and uric acid levels.[150,151]

Although weight loss may impact favorably on CHD risk factors, it is not clear that weight loss by itself alters CHD morbidity or mortality. However, decreased CHD mortality of overweight subjects with weight reduction to "acceptable" levels in both men and women for insurance purposes suggests a favorable effect.[152–154] However, potential biases in these data include unequal medical screening between weight loss and comparison groups, lack of control for smoking, and inadequate control for age.[155] The American Cancer Society's Cancer Prevention Study data were interpreted as showing modest reduction in CHD mortality with weight loss in some relative weight categories, but separate effects of voluntary and involuntary weight loss were not reported, and results were presented only for the broad age range 40 to 79 years.[156] Results of the British Regional Heart Study were reported as showing an 80% reduction in CHD mortality among overweight hypertensive men who achieved normal weight levels, but little effect on mortality in nonhypertensive obese men who lost weight.[157] These results apply only to effects of weight loss on premature mortality because of the relatively young age of the participants (40 to 59 years) and the short mortality follow-up period (4 years). In a review of six studies relating weight loss to longevity, the authors concluded that the evidence for a positive beneficial effect was equivocal.[156] Two studies did not provide data to support a positive effect, two studies found that mortality was actually increased in some subgroups, and only the biased life insurance studies supported a positive benefit. The authors noted that it would be difficult to ensure that the control group would not try to lose weight in a randomized trial, and suggested that careful observational studies would probably remain the most practical approach to this issue. In a subsequent 12-year follow-up of 43,457 overweight (BMI >30), never-smoking United States Caucasian women aged 40 to 64 years, age adjusted mortality data between those who intentionally lost weight were compared with data of those who had no change in weight.[158] In women with obesity-related health conditions, cardiovascular mortality was reduced only 9% by weight loss, with essentially no effect in those with no pre-existing illness. Thus beneficial effects on mortality with weight reduction may be observed in those with pre-existing CHD, but in the absence of established CHD, the benefit appears to be equivocal.

Summary and Conclusions

Recent estimates indicate that the prevalence of overweight in the United States adult population approximates one-third, while that in children and adolescents is about one-quarter. Most overweight children remain so as adults.

Epidemiological studies examining the relation between obesity and CHD mortality and morbidity have had conflicting results. A number of factors may contribute to these disparities, including misclassification due to imprecise measures of fatness, small cohort size and/or short term follow-up, failure to control for smoking, pre-existing disease, or physical activity, and inappropriate control for intermediate risk factors by which obesity may exert adverse effects. A major difficulty with interpretation of these studies revolves around the attempt to relate a single entity, itself conditioned by a variety of factors, to another complex interaction of factors conditioning CHD mortality and morbidity.

Large cohort population studies and/or those with longer follow-up indicate a predictive power for CHD mortality with maintenance BMI of >30 kg/m^2 for men, and >27 for women, which is less pronounced in older persons. However, excess total fat mass may have little effect on CHD mortality in selected sex, ethnic, social and racial groups, and extent of physical activity may condition mortality to a greater extent than obesity.

Almost all autopsy studies examining the relation between various indices of obesity and the extent and degree of coronary atheromatous disease have demonstrated no correlation, and a weak relation has occasionally been found. A recent large-scale multicenter study of younger persons, focusing on accidental deaths, and using both BMI and abdominal panniculus thickness to quantitate obesity, has demonstrated a correlation between obesity and atheromatous disease. However, the relation was obtained only in men with BMI > 30 kg/m^2, and there was no relation in women. Hypertension and dyslipidemia could not be critically evaluated. Very severe obesity is not associated with significant CHD on post-mortem examination. A number of studies demonstrate no correlation of arteriographic severity of CHD with indices of total fat mass. There are several studies indicating correlation of abdominal adiposity with extent of CHD on arteriogram, but there is no consensus, and in some the relation is lost when other factors are considered. Thus, cross-sectional anatomic studies provide virtually no support for an independent effect of excess total fat mass on the development or progression of the atheromatous process. Excess visceral abdominal adiposity may have some impact, but it is not clearly independent.

There is considerable evidence that excess abdominal visceral fat is associated with increased CHD mortality and morbidity. In subjects with this condition, particularly women, there tends to be a clustering of CHD risk factors, including dyslipidemia, NIDDM, hypertension, and hyperadrogenism. The incidence of these risk factors tends to increase steeply in most studies when the WHR is >1.0 in men, and >0.8 in women, with a monatomic correlation between increasing WHR and CHD mortality. Established CHD risk factors encountered with increased frequency in obese subjects include dyslipidemia, diabetes, hypertension, and hyperuricemia.

Plasma levels of triglycerides tend to rise and HDL levels tend to fall with increasing BMI, but the relation is not linear and there appears to be a BMI threshold of about 30 beyond which a plateau is observed. Total cholesterol and LDL serum level increases correlate less well with BMI. In addition central obesity is associated with a preponderance of the small dense LDL fraction, and increased concentrations of small VLDL. Although the incidence of NIDDM increases with incremental BMI, excess abdominal adiposity is more closely linked with glucose intolerance, hyperinsulinemia, insulin resistance, and lowered plasma HDL levels. While it is clear that excess total fat predisposes to hypertension, correlation of blood pressure with overweight is of a low order. The relation of elevated blood pressure levels to increasing BMI is stronger in children, young adults, and women than in men. Similarly, the increased incidence of hyperuricemia with obesity is not characterized by a clear correlation with increasing BMI.

From a public health standpoint it is noteworthy that there is a significant overrepresentation of CHD risk factors in children and adolescents with total body fat levels above 25% to 30%.

Multivariate analysis of epidemiological data has generally failed to indicate total fat mass as an independent predictor of CHD. Exceptions probably relate to misclassification or failure to account for one or more of the ever increasing number of CHD risk factors. Anatomical studies provide no consistent support for an effect of total fat mass on development or progression of the atheromatous process. Genetic sensitivity to CHD risk factors appears to be exacerbated by abdominal adiposity. Thus, the evidence at this time indicates that the effects of excess total and abdominal fat in relation to CHD are mediated through enhancement of atherogenic factors.

Sustained weight loss in obese subjects may be accompanied by significant reductions in plasma triglyceride levels, and elevations in HDL. Diminished abdominal adiposity may result in augmented LDL size. When glucose intolerance and hyperinsulinemia are present, weight loss brings about enhanced glucose oxidation, lower fasting insulin levels, and increased insulin sensitivity. Lowered blood pressure often occurs early after weight reduction with or without salt restriction in obese hypertensives. There is little correlation between decrements in weight and serum uric acid levels.

Whether the favorable impact of weight reduction in obese subjects on CHD risk factors translates into less CHD mortality and morbidity is not clear. There is some evidence to suggest a beneficial effect in those with pre-existing CHD.

References

1. Metropolitan Life Insurance Company: Metropolitan height and weight tables. *Stat Bull Metrop Ins Co* 64:2–9, 1983.
2. Kuczmarski RJ, Flegal KM, Campbell SM, et al: Increasing prevalence of

overweight among US adults. The national health and nutrition examination surveys 1960–1991. *JAMA* 272:205–21 1, 1994.

3. Gortmaker SL, Dietz WH, Sobol AM, et al: Increasing pediatric obesity in the United States. *Am J Dis Child* 141:535–540, 1987.

4. Epstein L: New developments in childhood obesity. In: Stunkard AI, Wadden TA (eds): *Obesity Theory and Therapy.* 2nd ed. Raven Press, New York, 1993, p. 301.

5. Bouchard C: Heredity and the path to overweight and obesity. *Med Sci Sports Exerc* 23:285–291, 1991.

6. Kvist H, Chowdhurty B, Grangard U, et al: Total and visceral adipose tissue volumes derived from measurements with computed tomography in adult men and women: Predictive equations. *Am J Clin Nutr* 48:1351–1361, 1988.

7. Stavig GR, Leonard AL, Igra A, et al: Indices of relative body weight and ideal weight charts. *J Chron Dis* 37:255–262, 1984.

8. Vague J: *Physiology of Adipose Tissue.* Excerpta Medica Foundation. Amsterdam. 1969.

9. Vernll D, Shoup E, Boyce L, et al: Recommended guidelines for body composition assessment in cardiac rehabilitation. *J Cardiopulm Rehab* 14:104–121, 1994.

10. Bouchard C, Bray GA, Hubbard VS: Basic and clinical aspects of regional fat distribution. *Am J Clin Nutr* 52:946–950, 1990.

11. Stallones RA: Epidemiologic studies of obesity. *Ann Intern Med* 103:1003–1005, 1985.

12. Barrett-Connor EL: Obesity, atherosclerosis, and coronary heart disease. *Ann Intern Med* 103:1010–1019, 1985.

13. Troiano RP, Frongillo EA Jr, Sobol I, Levitsky DA: The relationship between body weight and mortality: A quantitative analysis of combined information from existing studies. *Int J Obes* 20(suppl 4):109, 1996.

14. Manson JE, Stampfer MJ, Hennekins CH, Willett WC: Body weight and longevity. *JAMA* 257:353–358, 1987.

15. Sjostrom LV: Mortality of severely obese subjects. *Am J Clin Nutr* 55:516S–523S, 1992.

16. Borhani N0, Hechter HH, Breslow L: Report of a ten-year follow-up study of the San Francisco longshoremen. *J Chron Dis* 16:679–684, 1963.

17. Dyer AR, Stamler J, Berkson DL, et al: Relationship of relative weight and body mass index to 14-year mortality in the Chicago Peoples Gas Company Study. *J Chron Dis* 28:109–123, 1975.

18. Weinsier RL, Fuchs RJ, Kay TD, et al: Body fat: Its relationship to coronary heart disease, blood pressure, lipids, and other risk factors measured in a large male population. *Am J Med* 61:815–824, 1976.

19. Pelkonen R, Nikkila EA, Koskinen S, et al: Association of serum lipids and obesity with cariovascular mortality. *Br Med J* 2: 1185–1187, 1977.

20. Spawles R, Stamler J, Lindberg HA, et al: Asymptomatic hyperglycemia, and coronary heart disease in middle aged men in two employed populations in Chicago. *J Chron Dis* 32:805–815, I979.

21. Larsson B, Bjorntorp P, Tibblin G: The health consequences of moderate obesity. *Int J Obes* 5:97–116, 1981.

22. Lew EA, Garfinkel L: Variations in mortality by weight arnong 750,000 men and women. *J Chron Dis* 32:563–576, 1979.

23. Seidell JC, Verschureu, WMM, VanLeer EM, Kromhout D: Overweight, underweight, and mortality. *Arch Intern Med* 156:958–963, 1996.
24. Manson JE, Willett WC, Stampfer MJ, et al: Body weight and mortality among women. *N Engl J Med* 333:677–685, 1995.
25. Jousilahti P, Tuomilehto J, Vartiainen E, et al: Body weight, cardiovascular risk factors, and coronary mortality. *Circulation* 93:1372–1379, 1996.
26. Waaler HT: Height, Weight and Mortality: The Norwegian experience. *Acta Med Scand (Suppl)* 679:1–56, 1984.
27. Rissanen A, Heliovaara M, Knekt P, et al: Weight and mortality in Finnish men. *J Clin Epidermiol* 42:781–789, 1989.
28. Must A, Jacques PF, Dallal GE, et al: Long-term morbidity and mortality of overweight adolescents. A follow-up of the Harvard Growth Study of 1922–1935. *N Engl J Med* 327:1350–1355, 1992.
29. Keys A: Longevity of man: Relative weight and fatness in middle age. *Ann Med* 21:163–168, 1989.
30. Stevens J, Keil JE, Rust PF, et al: Body mass index and body girths as predictors of mortality in black and white women. *Arch Intern Med* 152:1257–1262, 1992.
31. Berlin JA, Colditz GA: A meta-analysis of physical activity in the prevention of coronary heart disease. *Am J Epidemiol* 132:612–628, 1990.
32. Stern M: Epidemiology of obesity and its link to heart disease. *Metabolism* 44(9 suppl 3):1–3, 1995.
33. Yater WM, Traum AH, Spring S, et al: Coronary artery disease in men eighteen to thirty nine years of age. *Am Heart J* 36:334–372, 1948.
34. Lee KT, Thomas WA: Relationship of body weight to acute myocardial infarction. *Am Heart J* 52:581–591, 1956.
35. Giertsen JC: Atherosclerosis in an autopsy series. *Acta Pathol Microbiol Scand* 67:305–321, 1966.
36. Bjurulf P: Atherosclerosis and body build. *Acta Med Scand* 349(Suppl): 1–99, 1959.
37. Ackerman RF, Dry TJ, Edwards JE: Relationship of various factors to the degree of coronary atherosclerosis in women. *Circulation* 1:1345–1354, 1950.
38. Wilkens RH, Roberts JC Jr, Moser C: Autopsy studies in atherosclerosis. *Circulation* 20:527–536, 1959.
39. Rhoades GG, Blackwelder WC, Stemmerman GN, et al: Coronary risk factors and autopsy findings in Japanese-American men. *Lab Invest* 38:304–311, 1978.
40. Montenegro MR, Solberg LA: Obesity, body weight, body length and atherosclerosis. *Lab Invest* 18:594–603, 1968.
41. Sternby NH: Atherosclerosis and body build. *Bull WHO* 53:601–604, 1976.
42. Solberg LA, Strong JP: Risk factors and atherosclerotic lesions: A review of autopsy studies. *Arteriosclerosis* 3:187–198, 1983.
43. Patel YC, Eggen DA, Strong JP: Obesity, smoking and atherosclerosis: A study of interassociations. *Atherosclerosis* 36:481–490, 1980.
44. Strong JP, Oalmann MC, Newman WP III, et al: Coronary heart disease in young black and white males in New Orleans: Community pathology study. *Am Heart J* 108:747–759, 1984.
45. McGill HC JR, McMahan CA, Malcolm GT, et al: Relation of glycohemoglobin and adiposity to atherosclerosis in youth. *Arterioscler Thromb Vasc Biol* 15:431–440, 1995.

46. Wilens SL: Bearing of general nutritional state on atherosclerosis. *Arch Intern Med* 79:129–147, 1947.
47. Amad KJ, Brennan JC, Alexander JK: The cardiac pathology of obesity. *Circulation* 32:740–745, 1965.
48. Alexander JK, Pettigrove JK: Obesity and congestive heart failure. *Geriatrics* 22:101–108, 1967.
49. Warnes CA, Roberts WC: The heart in massive (more than 300 pounds or 136 kilograms) obesity: Analysis of 12 patients studied at necropsy. *Am J Cardiol* 54:1087–1091, 1984.
50. Sorenson TIA, Sonne-Holm S: Mortality in extremely overweight young men. *J Chron Dis* 30:359–367, 1977.
51. Cramer K, Paulin S, Werko L: Coronary angiographic findings in correlation with age, body weight, blood pressure, serum lipids, and smoking habits. *Circulation* 33:888–900 1966.
52. Anderson AJ, Barboriak JJ, Rimm AA: Risk factors and angiographically determined coronary occlusion. *Am J Epidermiol* 107: 8–14, 1978.
53. Kramer JR, Matsuda Y, Mulligan JC, et al: Progression of coronary atherosclerosis. *Circulation* 63:519–526, 1981.
54. Hauner H, Stangl K, Schmatz C, et al: Body fat distribution in men with angiographically confirmed coronary artery disease. *Atherosclerosis* 85: 203–210, 1990.
55. Hartz A, Grubb B, Wild R, et al: The association of waist hip ratio and angiographically determined coronary artery disease. *Int J Obes* 14:657–665, 1990.
56. Hujamuta K, Toshima H, Koga Y, et al: Relationship between coronary risk factor and arteriographic feature of coronary atherosclerosis. *Jpn Circ J* 54.442–447,1990.
57. Reed D, Yano K: Predictors ofarteriographically defined coronary stenosis in the Honolulu Heart Program. *Am J Epidemiol* 134:111–122, 1991.
58. Zamboni M, Armellini F, Sheiban I, et al: Relation of body fat distribution in men and degree ofcoronary narrowings in coronary artery disease. *Am J Cardiol* 70:1135 1138, 1992.
59. Flynn MA, Cogg MN, Gibney MJ, et al: Indices ofobesity and body fat distribution in arteriographically defined coronary artery disease in men. *Irish J Med Sci* 162:503–509 1993.
60. Hodgson JM, Wahlquist N, Balazs NDH, Boxall JA: Coronary arteriosclerosis in relation to body fatness and its distribution. *Int J Obes Relat Metab Disord* 18:41–46, 1994.
61. Clark LT, Karve NM, Rones KT, et al: Obesity, distribution of body fat and coronary disease in black women. *Am J Cardiol* 73:895–896, 1994.
62. Morricone L, Ferrari M, Enrini R, et al: Angiographically determined coronary artery disease in relation to obesity and body fat distribution. *Int J Obes* 20(5uppl 4): 109, 1996.
63. Fuster V, Gotto AM Jr, Libby P, et al: Task Force I . Pathogenesis of coronary disease: The biologic role of risk factors. *J Am Coll Cardiol* 27:964–1047, 1996.
64. Buja LM, McAllister HA Jr: Coronary artery disease: Anatomic abnormalities. In: Willerson, JT, Cohn, JN (eds): *Cardiovascular Medicine.* Churchill Livingstone, New York, 1995, p. 316.
65. Larsson B, Svardsudd K, Welin L, et al: Abdominal adipose tissue distri-

bution, obesity, and risk of cardiovascular disease and death: A 13 year follow-up of participants in the study of men born in 1913. *Br Med J* 288:1401–1404, 1984.

66. Bjorntorp P, Sjostrum L: Adipose tissue dysfiznction and its consequences. In: Cryer A, Van R (eds): *New Prospective in Adipose Tissue.* Butterworths, London, 1984.

67. Donahue RP, Abbott RD, Bloom E, et al: Central obesity and coronary heart disease in men. *Lancet* 1:821–824, 1987.

68. Peiris AN, Sothmann MS, Hoffman RG, et al: Adiposity, fat distribution and cardiovascular risk. *Ann Intern Med* 110:867–872, 1989.

69. Bjorntorp P: Abdominal fat distribution and disease: An overview of epidemiological data. *Ann Med* 24:15–18, 1992.

70. Casassus P, Fontbonne A, Thibult N, et al: Upper body fat distribution: A hyperinsulinemia-independent predictor of coronary heart disease mortality— The Paris Prospective Study. *Arterioscler Thromb* 12: 1387–1392, 1992.

71. Bengtssom C, Bjorkelund C, Lapidus L, Lissner L: Associations of serum lipid concentrations and obesity with mortality in women: 20 year follow-up of participants in prospective population study in Gothenburg, Sweden. *Br Med J* 307:1385–1388, 1993.

72. Folsom AR, Kaye SA, Sellers TA, et al: Body fat distribution and 5-year risk of death in older women. *JAMA* 269:483–487, 1993.

73. Despres JP: Abdominal obesity as important component of insulin-resistance syndrome. *Nutrition* 9(5):452–459, 1993.

74. Wild RA: Obesity, lipids, cardiovascular risk, and androgen excess. *Am J Med* 98(1A):27S–325, 1995.

75. Croft JB, Keenan NL, Sheridan DP, et al: Waist-to-hip ratio in a biracial population: Measurement, implications, and cautions for using guidelines to deflne high risk for cardiovascular disease. *J Am Diet Assoc* 95(1): 60–64, 1995.

76. Bjontorp P: "Portal" adipose tissue as a generator of risk factors for cardiovascular disease and diabetes. *Arteriosclerosis* 10:493–496, 1990.

77. Bouchard C, Depres JP, Mauriege P: Genetic and non-genetic determinants of regional fat distribution. *Endocrinol Rev* 14:72–93, 1993.

78. Wilson PW: Established risk factors and coronary artery disease: The Framingham Study. *Am J Hypertens* 7(7):7S–12S, 1994.

79. Reeder BA, Angel A, Ledoux M, et al: Obesity and its relation to cardiovascular disease risk factors in Canadian adults. Canadian Heart Health Surveys Research Group. *Can Med Assoc J* 146(11):2009–2019, 1992.

80. Denke MA, Sempos CT, Grundy SM: Excess body weight: An under-recognized contributor to dyslipidemia in white American women. *Arch Intern Med* 154:401–410 1994.

81. Young TK, Gelskey DE: Is non-central obesity metabolically benign? Implications for prevention from a population survey. *JAMA* 274:1939–1941, 1995.

82. Barakat HΛ, Mooney N, O'Brien K, et al: Coronary heart disease risk factors in morbidly obese women with normal glucose tolerance. *Diabetes Care* 16(1):144–149, 1993 .

83. Teny RB, Wood PD, Haskell WL, et al: Regional adiposity pattern in relation to lipids, lipoprotein cholesterol, and lipoprotein subfraction mass in men. *J Clin Endocrinol Metab* 68:191–199, 1989.

84. Despres JP, Moorjani S, Ferland M, et al: Adipose tissue distribution and plasma lipoprotein levels in obese women: Importance of intra-abdominal fat. *Arteriosclerosis* 9:203–210, 1989.
85. Superko HR: New aspects of risk factors for the development of atherosclerosis, including small low-density lipoprotein, homocysteine, and lipoprotein(a). *Curr Opin Cardiol* 10:347–354, 1995.
86. Manson IE, Colditz GA, Stampfer MI, et al: A prospective study of maturity-onset diabetes mellitus and risk of coronary heart disease and stroke in women. *Arch Intern Med* 151(6):1141–1147, 1991.
87. National Institutes of Health Consensus Development Panel: Health implications of obesity. *Ann Intern Med* 103:1073–1077, 1985.
88. Pi-Sunyer FX: Health implications of obesity. *Am J Clin Nutr* 53(6 suppl):15955–16035, 1991.
89. Kissebah AH, Vydelingum M, Murray R, et al: Relation of body fat distribution to metabolic complications ofobesity. *J Clin Endocrinol Metab* 54:254–260, 1982.
90. Peiris AN, Mueller RA, Smith GA, et al: Splanchnic insulin metabolism in obesity. Influence of body fat distribution. *J Clin Invest* 78:1648–1657, 1986.
91. Wingard DL, Ferrara A, Barrett-Connor EL: Is insulin really a heart disease risk factor? *Diabetes Care* 18;1299–1304, 1995.
92. Despres JP, Lamarche B, Mauriege P, et al: Hyperinsulinemia as an independent risk factor for ischemic heart disease. *N Engl J Med* 334:952–957, 1996.
93. Laws A, Reaven GM: Evidence for an independent relationship between insulin resistance and fasting plasma HDL-cholesterol, triglyceride and insulin concentrations. *J Intern Med* 231:25–30, 1992.
94. Ostlund RE Jr, Staten M, Kohrt WM, et al: The ratio of waist-to-hip circumference, plasma insulin level, and glucose intolerance as independent predictors of the HDL_2 cholesterol level in older adults. *N Engl J Med* 322:229–234, 1990.
95. Stern MP: The insulin resistance syndrome: Controversy is dead, long live the controversy! *Diabetologia* 37:956–958, 1994.
96. Despres JP, Lamarche B, Dagenais GT: Letter to the editor. *N Engl J Med* 335:977, 1996.
97. Vijayaraghavan S, Hitman GA, Kopelman PG: Apolipoprotein-D polymorphism: A genetic marker for obesity and hyperinsulinemia. *J Clin Endocrinol Metab* 79(2):568–570, 1994.
98. Despres JP: Dyslipidaemia and obesity. *Baillieres Clin Endocrinol Metab* 8(3).029–000, 1994.
99. Nomori H, Horio H, Takagi M, et al: Clara cell protein correlation with hyperlipidemia. *Chest* 110:680–684, 1996.
100. Stamler R, Stamler I, Riedlinger WF, et al: Weight and blood pressure. Findings in hypertension screening of 1 million Americans. *JAMA* 240:1607–1610, 1978.
101. Voors AW, Webber LS, Frericks RR, Berenson GS: Body height and body mass as determinants of basal blood pressure in children. The Bogalusa Heart Study. *Am J Epidemiol* 106:101–108, 1977.
102. Johnson AL, Cornoni JC, Cassel JC, et al: Influence of race, sex, and weight on blood pressure behavior in young adults. *Am J Cardiol* 35:523–530, 1975.

103. Kannel WB, Brand N, Skinner J, et al: Relation of adiposity to blood pressure and development of hypertension: The Framingham Study. *Ann Intern Med* 67:48–59, 1967.
104. Hsu PH, Mathewson FAL, Rabkin SW: Blood pressure and body mass index patterns: A longitudinal study. *J Chron Dis* 30:93–113, 1977.
105. Court JM, Hill GJ, Dunlop M, et al: Hypertension in childhood obesity. *Austral Ped J* 10:296–300, 1974.
106. Alexander JK, Amad KH, Cole VW: Observations on some clinical features of extreme obesity with particular reference to cardiorespiratory effects. *Am J Med* 32:512–524, 1962.
107. Haynes RB: Is weight loss an effective treatment for hypertension? The evidence against. *Can J Physiol Pharmacol* 64:825–830, 1986.
108. MacMahon S, Cutlar J, Brittain E, et al: Obesity and hypertension: Epidemiological and clinical issues. *Eur Heart J* 8(Suppl B):57–70, 1987.
109. Williams DP, Going SB, Lohman TG, et al: Body fatness and risk for elevated blood pressure, total cholesterol, and serum lipoprotein ratios in children and adolescents. *Am J Public Health* 82(3):358–363, 1992.
110. Webber LS, Wattigney WA, Srinivasan AR, et al: Obesity studies in Bogalusa. *Am J Med Sci* 310(suppl):S53–S61, 1995.
111. Giddings SS, Bao W, Srinivasan AR, Berenson GS: Effects of secular trends in obesity on coronary risk factors in children: The Bogalusa Heart Study. *J Pediatr* 127:868–874, 1995.
112. Braddon F, Rodgers B, Wadsworth M, Davies J: Onset ofobesity in a 36 year birth cohort study. *Br Med J* 293:299–303, 1986.
113. Serdula N, Ivery D, Coates RJ, et al: Do obese children become obese adults? A review of the literature. *Prev Med* 22:167–177, 1993.
114. Guo SS, Roche AF, Chumlea WC, et al: The predictive value of childhood body mass index values for overweight at age 35. *Am J Clin Nutr* 59:810–819, 1994.
115. Gidding SS, Leibel RL, Daniels S, et al: Understanding obesity in youth. *Circulation* 94:3383–3387, 1996.
116. Levine W, Dyer AR, Skekelle RB, et al: Serum uric acid and 11.5 year mortality of middle-aged women. Findings of the Chicago Heart Association detection project in industry. *J Clin Epidemiol* 42:257–267, 1989.
117. Van Gaal L: Body fat mass distribution. Influence on metabolic and atherosclerotic parameters in non-insulin dependent diabetes and obese subjects with and without impaired glucose tolerance. *Verb K Acad Geneeskd Belg* 51(1):47–80, 1989. 118. Ernsberger P, Haskew P: Rethinking obesity, an alternative view of its health implications. *Obes Weight Regul* 6:57–137, 1987.
119. Hubert JW, Feinleib M, McNamara PM, Castelli WP: Obesity as an independent risk factor for cardiovascular disease: A 26-year follow-up of participants in the Framingham Heart Study. *Circulation* 67:968–977, 1983.
120. The Expert Panel II. Summary ofthe second report of the National Cholesterol Education Program (NCEP) expert panel on detection, evaluation, and treatment of high blood cholesterol in adults. *JAMA* 269:3015–3023, 1993.
121. Sjostrum LV: Morbidity of severely obese subjects. *Am J Clin Nutr* 55: 508S–515S, 1992.
122. Despres IP, Moorjam S, Lupien PJ, et al: Regional distribution of body fat,

plasma lipoproteins and cardiovascular disease. *Arteriosclerosis* 10:497–511, 1990.

123. Bouchard C, Despres JP, Mauriege P: Genetic and non-genetic determinants of regional fat distribution. *Endocr Rev* 14:72–93, 1993.

124. Dattilo Am, Kris-Etherton PM: Effects of weight reduction on blood lipids and lipoproteins: A meta-analysis. *Am J Clin Nutr* 56:320–328, 1992.

125. Palgi A, Read IL, Greenberg I, et al: Multidisciplinary treatment of obesity with a protein-sparing modified fast: Results in 668 outpatients. *Am J Public Health* 75:1190–1194, 1985.

126. Margolis S, Dobs AS: Nutritional management of plasma lipid disorders. *J Am Coll Nutr* 8(Suppl):33S–45S, 1989.

127. Kelly TM, Jones SB: Changes in serum lipids after gastric bypass surgery. Lack of a relationship to weight loss. *Int J Obes* 10(6):443–452, 1986.

128. Jimenez JG, Fong BS, Julien P, et al: Weight loss in massive obesity: Reciprocal changes in plasma HDL cholesterol and HDL binding to human adipocyte plasma membranes. *Metabolism* 37(6):580–586, 1988.

129. Gleysteen IJ, Barboriak JI, Sasse EA: Sustained coronary-risk-factor reduction after gastric bypass for morbid obesity. *Am J Clin Nutr* 51(5):774–778, 1990.

130. Brolin RE, Kenler HA, Wilson AC, et al: Serum lipids after gastric bypass surgery for morbid obesity. *Int J Obes* 14(11):939–950, 1990.

131. Barakat HA, Carpenter JW, McLendon VD, et al: Influence of obesity, impaired glucose tolerance, and NIDDM on LDL structure and composition. Possible link between hyperinsulinemia and atherosclerosis. *Diabetes* 39(12):1527–1533, 1990.

132. Svendsen OL, Hassger C, Christiansen C: Effect of an energy-restrictive diet, with or without exercise, on lean tissue mass, resting metabolic rate, cardiovascular risk factors, and bone in overweight postmenopausal women. *Am J Med* 95(2):131–140, 1993.

133. Wood PD, Stefanick N, Williams PT, Haskell WL: The effects on plasma lipoproteins of a prudent weight-reducing diet, with or without exercise, in overweight men and women. *N Engl J Med* 325(7):461–466, 1991.

134. Wabitsch M, Hauner H, Heinze E, et al: Body-fat distribution and changes in atherogenic risk-factor profile in obese adolescent girls during weight reduction. *Am J Clin Nutr* 60(1):54–60, 1994.

135. Fox AA, Thompson IL, Butterfield GE, et al : Effects of diet and exercise on common cardiovascular disease risk factors in moderately obese older women. *Am J Clin Nutr* 63(2):225–233, 1996.

136. Newburgh LH: Control of hyperglycemia of obese diabetics by weight reduction. *Ann Intern Med* 17:935–942, 1942.

137. Bagdade ID, Porte D Jr, Brunzell JD, et al: Basal and stimulated hyperinsulinism: Reversible metabolic sequelae of obesity. *J Lab Clin Med* 83:563–569, 1974.

138. Franssila A, Rissanen A, Ekstrand A, et al: Effects of weight loss on substrate oxidation, energy expenditure, and insulin sensitivity in obese individuals. *Am J Clin Nutr* 55:356–361, 1992.

139. Tochikubo 0, Miyajima E, Okabe K, et al: Improvement of multiple coronary risk factors in obese hypertensives by reduction of intra-abdominal fat. *Jpn Heart J* 35(6):715–725, 1994.

140. Ellahou HE, Jania A, Gaon T, et al: Body weight reduction necessary to

attain normotension in the overweight hypertensive patient. *Int J Obes* 5(Suppl 1):157–163, 1981.

141. Rissanen A, Pietinen P, Siljamaki-Oransuu U, et al: Treatment of hypertension in obese subjects: Efficacy and feasibility of weight and salt reduction programs. *Acta Med Scand* 218:149–156, 1985.

142. Reisin E: Weight reduction in the management of hypertension: Epidemiologic and mechanistic evidence. *Clin J Physiol Pharmacol* 64:818–824, 1986.

143. Goldstein DJ: Beneficial effects of modest weight loss. *Int J Obes Metab Disord* 16:397–415, 1992.

144. Sowers JK, Nyby M, Stern N, et al: Blood pressure and hormone changes associated with weight reduction in the obese. *Hypertension* 4:686–691, 1982.

145. Cohen N, Flamenbaum W: Obesity and hypertension. Demonstration of a "floor" effect. *Am J Med* 80:177–181, 1986.

146. Sabotte D, Stunkard AJ: The effects of weight reduction on blood pressure in 301 obese subjects. *Arch Intern Med* 150:1701–1704, 1990.

147. Reisin E, Abel R, Modan M, et al: Effect of weight loss without salt restriction on the reduction in blood pressure in overweight hypertensive patients. *N Engl J Med* 298: 1–6, 1978.

148. Staessen J, Fagard R, Lijnen P, Amery A: Body weight, sodium intake and blood pressure. *J Hypertens* 7(suppl 1):S19-S23, 1989.

149. Weinsier RL, James LD, Darnell BE, et al: Obesity-related hypertension: Evaluation of the separate effects energy restriction and weight reduction on hemodynamic and neuroendocrine status. *Am J Med* 90(4):460–468, 1991.

150. Ashley FW Jr, Kannel WB : Relation of weight changes to changes in atherogenic traits: The Framingham Study. *J Chron Dis* 27:103–114, 1974.

151. Krizek V: Serum uric acid in relation to body weight. *Ann Rheum Dis* 25: 456–458, 1966.

152. Dublin LI: Relation of obesity to longevity. *N Engl J Med* 248:971–974, 1953.

153. Shephard WP, Marks HH: Life insurance looks at the arteriosclerosis problem. *Minn Med* 38:736–742, 1955.

154. Society of Actuaries: *Build and Blood Pressure Study.* Vol 1, Chicago, 1959.

155. Williamson DF, Pamuk ER: The association between weight loss and longevity. A review of the evidence. *Ann Intern Med* 119:731–736, 1993.

156. Hammond EC, Garfinkle L: Coronary heart disease, stroke, and aortic aneurysm. *Arch Environ Health* 19:167–182, 1969.

157. Wannamethee G, Sharpe AG: Weight change in middle-aged British men: Implications for health. *Eur J Clin Nutr* 44:133–142, 1990.

158. Williams DF, Pamuk E, Thun M, et al: Prospective study of intentional weight loss and mortality in never-smoking overweight US white women aged 40–64 years. *Am J Epidemiol* 141:1128–1141, 1995.

159. Borntorp P: Fatty acids, hyperinsulinemia, and insulin resistance: Which comes first? *Curr Opin Lipidol* 5:166–174, 1994.

Appendix

Quantification of Obesity

Several indices have been utilized to quantitate the degree of obesity. Relative body weight, also known as Metropolitan relative weight and percent of ideal body weight, is based on the extent to which the observed body weight surpasses ideal body weight as predicted from height and gender.[1] Relative body weight (%) is calculated by dividing actual body weight by ideal body weight and then multiplying the quotient by 100. Obesity is generally considered to be mild when relative body weight lies between 120% and 150% of ideal, and severe when body weight exceeds 150% of ideal. The term morbid obesity has been used interchangeably with severe obesity, but is more commonly applied to those whose actual body weight is twice their ideal body weight or more. The term percent overweight has been used in some studies to quantify obesity. Percent overweight is the percentage over and above ideal body weight. For example, a patient whose actual body weight is twice ideal body weight would be 100% overweight. The severity of obesity can also be quantified using other indices based on height and weight,[2] which largely relate to total adipose tissue mass. One such index is the ratio of body weight to height (BW/Ht). There is a linear relation between BW/Ht and body weight expressed as percent ideal; values of 0.6, 0.8, and 1.0 kg/cm correspond to body weights of approximately 150%, 200%, and 250% ideal, respectively.[3] Another is the body mass index (BMI), calculated as the quotient of body weight in kilograms and height in meters squared. See Table 1 for BMI categories.

From: Alpert MA, and Alexander JK, (eds). *The Heart and Lung in Obesity*. Armonk, NY: Futura Publishing Company, Inc., © 1998.

Table 1
Body Mass Index Categories

Categories	Body Mass Index (kg/m²)
Acceptable Range (low disease risk/mortality)	20.0–25.0
Mildly Overweight (Increased disease risk/mortality)	25.1–27.0
Moderately Overweight/Obese	27.1–30.0
Markedly Overweight/Obese	30.1–40.0
Morbidly Obese	> 40.0

(Reproduced with permission from Reference 18.)

Amount and Distribution of Body Fat

Amount of body fat can be assessed in a number of ways, including anthropometric analysis, body density from underwater weight, isotopic techniques to determine body water or body potassium, dual-photon absorptiometry, bioimpedance analysis, and total body electrical conductivity.[4] Body fat comprises approximately 15% to 20% of body mass in healthy men,[5] and 25% to 30% in healthy women.[6] With obesity, body fat typically comprises 40% to 45%, but can represent as much as 60% or more of body mass.[6] Because of logistic considerations, equipment expense, and degree of tester training and experience needed, these modalities have been largely reserved for research study, being poorly adapted to large scale epidemiological surveys. Measurement of skinfold thicknesses is an economical and reasonably accurate technique for assessment of body composition, but provides only an estimate of subcutaneous fat deposits. The Jackson/Pollock generalized formulas for skinfold measurements at three body sites, which is a commonly used technique, is highly correlated with body densitometry measurements.[7] Subscapular skinfold thickness has been shown to correlate with total fat mass,[8] percent body fat[8] and intra-abdominal fat.[9] However, BMI or waist/height ratios may be modalities better suited for applicability with markedly obese patients in whom accuracy of regression equations declines, and anatomic sites may be difficult to locate or hard to palpate.

The waist/hip ratio (WHR) has been used as a surrogate measurement of abdominal visceral adipose tissue volume, and is superior to BMI in this regard.[10] This ratio is obtained by dividing the abdominal circumference measurement as the smallest below the rib cage above the umbilicus by the largest circumference at buttock level or below the pelvic brim. "Ideal" WHR levels have been appraised to be 0.90 or less for men, and 0.80 or less for women. For more precise assessment of abdominal visceral fat, ultrasonography,[11] computed tomography,[12] or magnetic resonance imaging[13, 14] have been used.

Fat-Free Mass

Obesity is associated with increases in fat-free mass (FFM), body cell mass, and total body water as well as increased fat mass and body weight.[15] The percent of fat increases curvilinearly with BMI, such that % fat = (BMI − 16.1) × 65.7/BMI in men and % fat = (BMI − 13.8) × 75.7/BMI in women.[16] From these data it can be calculated that FFM/body weight = 3.60 $\text{BMI}^{-0.480}$ in men and FFM/body weight = 3.87 $\text{BMI}^{-0.549}$ in women (Figure 1). To put this into perspective, a male with body weight of 70 kg and BMI 23 kg/m² would have a FFM of 56 kg, but if his weight increased to 105 kg, BMI would be 34.5 kg/m² and his FFM would increase to 69 kg. In other words, 63% of the weight gain is fat and 37% is FFM. The resting energy expenditure is proportional

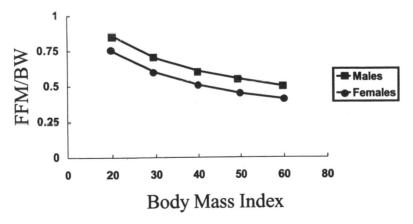

Figure 1. Ratio of fat-free mass to body weight (FFM/BW) as a function of BMI in males (filled square) and females (filled circles). Data from Gray and Fujioka[16] have been recalculated to obtain equations FFM/BW = 3.60 $\text{BMI}^{-0.48}$ for males and FFM/BW = 3.85 $\text{BMI}^{-0.549}$ for females.

Table 2
Indices of Body Weight in Normals (NL), Obese Subjects (OB),
and Obesity Hypoventilation Syndrome (OHS).

Variable	Units	NL	OB	OHS
BW	(kg)	72	127	131
BW	(% ideal)	105	195	201
BW/Ht	(kg/cm)	0.42	0.75	0.78
BMI	(kg/m^2)	24	45	46

BW = body weight; Ht = height; BMI = body mass index (see text).

to the FFM and body cell mass, and the ratio of resting energy expenditure to FFM is the same in mild and severe obesity as it is in normal weight subjects.[15,17]

Table 2 summarizes typical values of various parameters and indices for quantifying obesity, for normal subjects and for patients with morbid obesity and those with the obesity-hypoventilation syndrome (OHS). Values in OHS are nearly identical to those in simple obesity. However, it seems likely that there is relatively more fat and less muscle in OHS, because OHS patients are sicker and less active.

References

1. Metropolitan Life Insurance Company. *Stat Bull* 40:1–4, 1959.
2. Seltzer F: Measurement of overweight. *Stat Bull* 65:20–23, 1984.
3. Ray CS, Sue DY, Bray G, et al: Effects of obesity on respiratory function. *Am Rev Resp Dis* 128:501–506, 1983.
4. Pierson RNJ, Wang J, Heymsfield SB, et al: Measuring body fat: Calibrating the rulers. Intermethod comparison of 389 normal Caucasian subjects. *Am J Physiol* 261:E103-E108, 1991.
5. Norgan NG, Durnin JVGA: The effect of 6 weeks of overfeeding on the body weight, body composition, and energy metabolism of young men. *Am J Clin Nutr* 33:978–988, 1990.
6. Morse WI, Soeldner JS: The non-adipose body mass of obese women: Evidence of increased muscularity. *Can Med Assoc J* 90:723–725, 1964.
7. Jackson AS, Pollock ML: Practical assessment of body composition. *Phys Sportsmed* 13:76–90, 1985.
8. Chumlea WC, Roche AF, Webb P: Body size, subcutaneous fatness and total body fat in older adults. *Int J Obes* 8:311–317, 1984.
9. Peiris A, Hennes M, Evans DJ, et al: Relationship of anthropometric mea-

surements of body fat distribution to the metabolic profile in pre-menopausal women. *Acta Med Scand* 723(suppl 1):179–188, 1988.

10. Despres J-P, Prudhomme D, Poulist MC, et al: Estimation of deep abdominal adipose-tissue accumulation from simple anthropometric measurements in men. *Am J Clin Nutr* 54:471–477, 1991.

11. Suzuki R, Watanabe S, Hirai Y, et al: Abdominal wall fat index, estimated by ultrasonography for assessment of the ratio of visceral fat to subcutaneous fat in the abdomen. *Am J Med* 95:309–314, 1993.

12. Busetto L, Baggio MB, Zurlo F, et al: Assessment of abdominal fat distribution in obese patients: Anthropometry versus computerized tomography. *Int J Obes* 16:731–736, 1992.

13. Sobol W, Rossner S, Hinson B, et al: Evaluation of a new magnetic resonance imaging method for quantitating adipose tissue areas. *Int J Obes* 15:589–599, 1991.

14. Ross R, Shaw KD, Rissanen J, et al: Sex differences in lean and adipose tissue distribution by magnetic resonance imaging: Anthropometric relationships. *Am J Clin Nutr* 59:1277–1285, 1994.

15. Verga S, Buscemi C, Caimi G: Resting energy expenditure and body composition in morbidly obese, obese and control subjects. *Acta Diabetologica* 31:47–51, 1994.

16. Gray DS, Fiuioka K: Use of relative weight and body mass index for the determination of obesity. *J Clin Epidemiol* 44:545–550, 1991.

17. Leibel RL, Rosenbaum M, Hirsch J: Changes in energy expenditure resulting from altered body weight. *N Engl J Med* 332:621–628, 1995.

18. Verrill D, Shoup E, Boyce L, et al: Recommended guidelines for body composition assessment in cardiac rehabilitation. *J Cardiopulm Rehabil* 14:104–121, 1994.

Index

245